Reclaiming Your Sexual Self

How You Can Bring
Desire Back into Your Life

Kathryn Hall, Ph.D.

WILEY

John Wiley & Sons, Inc.

Published by John Wiley & Sons, Inc., Hoboken, New Jersey
Published simultaneously in Canada

For general information about our other products and services, please contact our
Customer Care Department within the United States at (800) 762-2974, outside the
United States at (317) 572-3993 or fax (317) 572-4002.

Wiley also publishes its books in a variety of electronic formats. Some content that
appears in print may not be available in electronic books. For more information
about Wiley products, visit our web site at www.wiley.com.

Library of Congress Cataloging-in-Publication Data:
Hall, Kathryn.
    Reclaiming your sexual self : how you can bring desire back into your
life / Kathryn Hall.
        p.   cm.
    Includes bibliographical references and index.
    ISBN 0-471-27427-5 (pbk.)
    1. Sex.   2. Hygiene, Sexual.   3. Sex customs.   I. Title.
HQ21.H31355   2004
306.7—dc22

2004006064

10   9   8   7   6   5   4   3

This book is about passion and connection.
This book is dedicated to Jim,
who constantly affirms the importance of both.

Contents

Acknowledgments

I am greatly indebted to the women and men who have trusted me to be their therapist and who have shared with me their lives, their loves, their pains, and their pleasures. It was always a journey of mutual discovery. They were and are my best teachers. I have also been fortunate to have friends and colleagues who have listened to me as I struggled with the ideas that have ultimately formed the basis of this book. To those who read all or parts of the manuscript and offered their comments, advice, and always constructive ideas, I am particularly thankful: Gerianne Alexander, Linda Courey, Darson Hall, Cynthia Graham, Phyllis Marganoff, Jim Mastrich, Myron Pawliw, Claire Tondreau, and Gerald Wiviott. My brilliant editor, Lisa Considine, helped translate what happens in a private therapy hour to the pages of this book. Her insights, intelligence, patience, and unfailing support and encouragement got me through some sleepless nights. I first brought the idea of this book to the woman who became my agent, Carol Mann. Her help in getting this book out of my head and into the hands of publishers was invaluable. Thanks also go to Elizabeth Zack, who acquired this book for John Wiley & Sons. From the bottom of my heart, I thank my sons, Zachary and Devin, who had to hear "Wait" a few times too many while I was writing this book. I am extraordinarily grateful to the mothers and fathers of Lambertville, New Jersey, where I make my home, for being "the village" and helping to care for my boys when they could "wait" no longer. My most heartfelt thanks and gratitude go to my husband, Jim Mastrich, who believed I could and would write this book, even when I did not. Above all he provides me with the inspiration and motivation to be passionate in my life.

Introduction

The sheer number of women disinterested in sex tells us that something is wrong. The latest estimates indicate that approximately one-third of adult women are not really interested in sex.[1] One might wonder whether the sex available to these women is really worth being interested in. One might wonder what else is going on in the lives of these women that is either more interesting than sex or that is more demanding of their time and attention. But instead of looking at what might cause so many women to feel sexually disenfranchised, 33 million women are being told that there is something wrong with *them*. And without any evidence of a physical malady, many of these women have accepted the label of "sexually dysfunctional."

True, there are some physical conditions that can cause or contribute to low sexual desire. But it defies logic to believe that a third of all women suffer from low testosterone, restricted blood flow to the genitals, or a chemical imbalance in the brain. Nevertheless, the fact remains that a great deal of money is to be made if women believe that the answer to their desire woes can be found in a pill or a patch. Instead of blaming women or finding fault with our biological makeup, I suggest we explore other explanations for this epidemic sexual ennui.

My Story: The Asexual Sex Therapist

After the birth of my second child, I had no sexual desire for quite some time. I was tired, stressed out, and felt pulled in several different directions at the same time. Everyone seemed to want more from

1

me—my children, my husband, my friends, and, my patients. And it was during this time, in my professional circles, that I encountered the experts. Something must happen, they surmised, to the hormone levels of women after the birth of their second child, because many women lose sexual interest at that time. Hearing this, I felt the anger rising within me. These experts had no evidence (and still don't) of any hormonal changes, and the conclusions they jumped to made it obvious that they weren't raising two children. These same experts were writing books, going on talk shows, and reaching out to professionals like myself to advocate Viagra and testosterone for sexually disinterested women. "Why not just give us amphetamines," I grumbled to myself, "so we can keep going around the clock?" It was then I knew I didn't need testosterone—I needed sleep. I didn't want Viagra—I wanted help with all the things I was trying to juggle. It finally dawned on me that trying to have the same level of involvement in my work, in my marriage, and with my three-year-old as I'd had before a new infant was in my life was an enterprise doomed to failure. Something had to give. My absent sexual desire should have been a signal to me that my life was out of balance. I needed to make changes in my life to accommodate the new demands of being a mother to two children. So instead of trying to do it all, I began to do things differently. I said no to additional responsibilities at home and work. I traded favors with friends and hired baby-sitters. I asked more of my husband. When I was finally able to see beyond the overwhelming responsibilities that come with motherhood, I discovered a very powerful aphrodisiac: the sight of my husband changing diapers, playing with our sons, preparing strained vegetables, or vacuuming the playroom. With time for myself, and time with my body to myself, I was able to be a sexual woman once again.

My own experience made me realize two things. The first is that the so-called sex experts know very little about sexual desire in women. Neither my sex therapy training nor my readings in the field prepared me for my own experience. There was no mention of the therapeutic value of having one's husband do housework or child care. There were only sexual exercises to be done together or alone, which I had neither the time for nor the interest in. The second realization I had was how completely I had bought into the myth that women can have it all—a career, an emotionally and sexually fulfilling relationship, and talented, intelligent, well-mannered children who are a constant joy to nurture, stimulate, and educate. The most damaging part of the myth is that I believed I could have all this if I just worked hard enough to get it. Expert advice that promotes the belief that there's something wrong with you if you don't "have it all" ignores the reality of many women's life situations. In my own case, there was nothing wrong with my hormone levels. My lack of desire was appropriate to my situation. When I changed the situation, my desire returned, although not in the same manifestation as when I was younger and single. My personal experience prompted me to reexamine and question many of the prevailing theories about female sexuality and sexual desire. This book is the product of that journey and the resultant success I have had helping my clients to reclaim their sexual selves.

Expert Opinions

Frankly, it appears that most sex experts have just taken it for granted that people want to have sex. Just look at the titles of the self-help books: *Hot Monogamy, Extended Massive Orgasm, How to Have Magnificent Sex,* and *The Joy of Sex,* to name a few. All these books assume that the reader wants to have sex; actually the authors assume that the reader wants to have great sex, a lot. Women with low sexual desire will not find much help in these books. When a woman consults an expert, the goal of the consultation is to discover what is inhibiting her desire. No one ever asks why her partner wants to have sex. Imagine a sex therapist turning to your husband and asking, "But why do you want to have sex with your wife when you can see that she is tired, stressed out, and completely disinterested? Exactly *what* is turning you on at those times?" It's unimaginable, because the desire to have sex is assumed to be innate and healthy, and the context in which it occurs is rarely considered (unless of course the context is totally inappropriate, as it is in cases of rape and child abuse).

Because the study of human sexual behavior grew out of the study of animal behavior and reproduction, there has always been a strong emphasis on the sex drive. Sex researchers believed that the goal of the human sex drive was twofold: facilitating both reproduction and the bond between two people that would ensure the survival of their offspring. Women were said to be attracted to strong men who could protect them and their children from danger. What "strong" meant evolved from physical to financial ability. Men were said to be attracted to young and fertile women. Furthermore, because men would want to have as many offspring as possible to ensure the survival of their own gene pool, they were said to have stronger sex drives. Monogamy was therefore assumed to be more difficult for men than for women.

Despite the fact that there is little evidence for these theories and that the theories themselves are disputed among scholars, many people believe in the truth of this biological/evolutionary perspective. It makes sense to them and explains behavior they observe. There is a general acceptance of the existence of a sex drive, with "drive" defined as a powerful need or instinct that motivates behavior. This idea of a sex drive brings with it the assumption that sex is natural and does not need or require special effort. Social values have dictated how the sex drive should or should not be expressed, but it is always a given that it is there.

Freud brought the biological-drive theory of sex into psychiatry. He used the word "libido" to denote the life force, which he assumed was an inborn, biological, sexual energy. Women who were not interested in sex or who did not enjoy sex were assumed to have something psychologically wrong with them. The label "frigid," applied to women who did not enjoy or desire sex, was used also to describe a personality type (cold, unfeeling), and people came to believe that the personality caused the lack of sexual passion. Psychiatrists, following Freud's lead, traditionally viewed women's sexual disinterest as a symptom of a deeper psychological problem or inner conflict. Again the underlying assumption is that sexual desire is natural, and if it is lacking, there must be something wrong with the individual. Psychiatry looked for inner conflicts and paid little attention to the context in which sex occurred (an individual's life circumstances, the quality of the marriage and/or sexual relationship).

Sex Therapy

Masters and Johnson were pioneers in sex research and came to public attention with their 1966 book, *Human Sexual Response*.[2] As medical professionals, they actually solicited volunteers who agreed to have their bodily responses (such as pulse, skin temperature, respiration) monitored as they had sex. While it had been assumed that men's and women's sexualities were fundamentally different, Masters and Johnson argued that male and female sexual responses were remarkably similar. Women's arousal was observed to be somewhat slower to peak than men's, but apart from speed, the pattern of responding was similar. According to Masters and Johnson, the human sexual response cycle could be divided into four separate phases: arousal, plateau, orgasm, and resolution. Sexual problems were problems that men and women experienced in each of these phases. Erection problems in men or lubrication difficulties in women were specific to the arousal and plateau phases. Difficulties with ejaculation or orgasms were problems of the orgasm phase.

Remarkably, sexual desire was not included as part of the sexual response cycle, nor was lack of desire considered to be a problem on its own. If someone did not want to have sex, Masters and Johnson believed that there must be another sexual problem, such as difficulty having orgasm or experiencing pain with intercourse, that was responsible. In other words, the only reason someone would not want to have sex was if the sex was not worth wanting.

Masters and Johnson's research gave birth to sex therapy, a distinct brand of psychotherapy that was focused on treating the sexual problems they had identified. Their focus on behavior and instruction is what set this approach apart from traditional "talk therapies." In a typical Masters and Johnson–style sex therapy clinic, a couple was interviewed about their sexual relationship and then given exercises to do at home that would help them overcome their sexual difficulties. Anxiety about sexual performance was thought to be the most common cause of sexual dysfunction.

By the mid-1970s, the number of sex therapy clinics was growing. It was in the seventies that the number of complaints from people regarding sexual desire became apparent. These people did not suffer from another sexual problem, as Masters and Johnson had thought. When sex got going, it was good. It was just that they never or rarely felt like having sex. One of the first to identify low sexual desire as a distinct issue was Helen Singer Kaplan, a psychiatrist and sex therapist. Like other sex experts, Dr. Kaplan viewed sexual desire as an innate urge, but she also theorized that we have sexual suppressors or brakes that provide control of our sexual appetites. Dr. Kaplan believed that healthy sexual desire was blocked when men and women focused on their partner's negative qualities and ignored the positive aspects.

Since Masters and Johnson and Helen Singer Kaplan, sex therapists have come to assume that healthy or normal sexuality involves the ability to block out "distractions" that would lead to performance anxiety or low desire. So if a woman complained that her husband's or boyfriend's surly behavior was a turnoff, she was told to leave her anger at the bedroom door. She was told to stop thinking about the negative and to concentrate instead on the physical sensations resulting from sexual touch. If her partner didn't really excite her, she was told to fantasize, even about someone else. If a relationship was really bad, a couple was sent to marriage counseling. Sex therapy dealt with sex, as if sex could be separated from the entirety of one's life.

Hormone Replacement?

Sex research, which informs and influences the treatment of sexual problems, largely continues to regard sexual desire as an innate drive that, if deficient, indicates a problem within an individual. However, sex research is now heavily funded and sponsored by drug companies, who have provided the resources that the more conservative and financially strapped government agencies could not. The result is that we are now looking at what is biologically or biochemically wrong with women who have little desire for sex—in other words, what a pill could correct.

If sex therapists have been telling women to be more like men in their ability to focus on sexual pleasure to the exclusion of all else, the pharmaceutical industry is pushing women to be more hormonally like men. The problem, as the drug companies define it, is that women are deficient in the hormone of desire, also known as the male hormone, testosterone.

Women are being bombarded with the message that hormones are responsible for sexual desire. Testosterone, progesterone, estrogen, and prolactin are the hormones that are or have been the major focus of study. It is true that in order to have good sexual and reproductive functioning, women need certain minimal amounts of these hormones. But the fact that women need some amount of some of these hormones to have sexual desire does not mean that lack of sexual desire necessarily indicates a hormonal problem. Indeed, it would be quite shocking to believe that 33 million American women suffer hormonal abnormalities. To date there are no studies that show that hormonal levels are different in women with low desire versus those with high desire. Nevertheless, where women once bristled at the idea that because of their hormonal cycles they were emotionally unfit for many traditionally male occupations and pursuits, women now wear their hormonal lability like a badge of honor. It gives them a reason to be angry and irritable: "I'm just PMS-ing!" It takes away the blame felt for sexual disinterest: "My hormones are out of whack!" But as Dr. Christiane Northrup explains in her book *The Wisdom of Menopause,*[3] hormones do not exist in a universe of their own. Your hormonal fluctuations may make you more or less sensitive to things that are nonetheless real issues in your life. If just prior to your period you find yourself bursting into tears because your husband left the toilet seat up (again), his inattention to things that are important to you is likely to be a real issue in your relationship. While you may otherwise just sigh and shrug off your partner's behavior, you can use your heightened sensitivity to recognize and respond to small problems in your life before they become big problems with a history of buried resentment.

The authors of the National Life and Health Survey, whose data were used to promote the idea that women's sexual problems have reached epidemic proportions, note, "If sex were only a matter of hormones, our data would make little sense. On average, sex hormone levels are not much changed until age fifty, although by age thirty people are already having less frequent partnered sex."[4]

The important point to be made here is that hormone levels are not solely responsible for our sexual desires or our sexual disinterest, nor should we aspire to have hormone cocktails to override our natural inclinations.

Listening to Our Sexual Selves

Our sexual feelings provide us with important information about the nature and quality of our life and our relationships. We need to listen to and learn from these feelings, not ignore or deny them. When sexual desire wanes, we have to attend to the message inherent in this change. Is there a physical problem, or more likely is there something else in our life or relationship that is not working? Sometimes traditional medicine promotes an adversarial relationship with our bodies. Often the body is viewed as having a problem that must be fought. While it may be appropriate to talk of fighting cancer, we cannot "fight" low sexual desire in the same way. What is it that we are supposed to be attacking?

In this book I have endeavored to put sexual desire into context— the reality of women's lives. We are physical beings to be sure, but our sexual interest depends upon much more than hormones and blood flow. So while I will discuss the possible physical bases for sexual desire problems, the remainder of the book looks beyond the corporal. A lack of desire means that something is out of balance in our lives, our relationships, and our sexuality. After discovering the source of your sexual disinterest, you will be given the tools to increase your sexual desire, methods I have successfully used in my clinical practice of sex therapy. This is not a one-size-fits-all or quick-fix approach but a method to bring desire back into the unique circumstances of your life and keep it there for good.

1

Sex Doesn't Exist in a Vacuum

I think about sex a lot. It is on my mind the first thing in the morning, and it is invariably the last thing I think about at night. Every morning I get up and say to myself that today I will have sex with my husband; I will do it. By noon I can feel my resolve waning, and by evening I am feeling so stressed that sex is out of the question. The laundry, the bills, the household chores—they all seem so much more important, so much more urgent than spending time alone with my husband. In the past I got away with this, but now my husband gets really angry and even threatens to leave. I love my husband. I wish I wanted to have sex, but I just don't. If I don't get my desire back, I may lose him.

—Anna

Anna is not unusual. A surprising number of women feel little or no sexual desire. In a recent, large-scale national survey, one-third of the women surveyed said they were simply not interested in sex.[1] That corresponds to some 33 million women in the United States alone! Some women have never felt very excited about sex and have never really been very sexual. Others, like Anna, previously enjoyed a high level of sexual interest, only to have their passion fade at some point in their lives.

Feeling asexual in a sexual world is a difficult and alienating experience. It's like living in a foreign country and not speaking the language or being the only one not getting the joke. Most people don't understand how upsetting it is to lack sexual passion for someone you love. While men can also experience diminished sexual desire, the partners of women with low or absent desire often believe that their wives or girlfriends have it just the way they want it. These men may complain of feeling manipulated, used, controlled, and even castrated. The truth is that women care very much about the quality of their intimate relationships and they care very much about the welfare and well-being of those they love. The loss of sexual passion is very distressing to most women. Women do not want to let their partners down, nor do they want to feel that they are past their sexual prime. The anger, the bitterness, and the constant battles about sex can wreak havoc in even the best of relationships.

How Much Is Enough?

The pressure to have sex that many women feel in their intimate relationships is supported by our society's emphasis on sex and bolstered by the belief that everyone else wants to have sex, loves having sex, and is having more sex and better sex than we are. The National Health and Life Survey[2] reported that approximately one-half of couples who are married or living together have sex twice a week or more. Yet despite the frequency with which couples have sex, remember that about one-third of women report that they have little interest in it. A lack of desire does not necessarily mean a lack of sex. Despite the large percentage of women who said that they were not interested in sex, fewer than 3 percent of women living with a husband or a boyfriend abstained from sex during that same time period. The vast majority of partnered women are having sex several times a month or more, if they are interested or not. What may be most predictive of the frequency of a woman's sexual activity is her partner's sexual interest, not her own.

Frankly, we don't really have a way of measuring sexual desire. We know clearly when it is not there, and we believe we know when it is excessive. Women who appear too interested in sex, who have too much sex, or who enjoy sex too much are labeled nymphomaniacs. Women who have little interest in sex or who appear not to enjoy it are labeled frigid. What's acceptable? What's just right?

These questions presume that there is an optimum level of sexual interest. But this optimum amount keeps changing according to societal beliefs and the expectations of our partners. What is optimal for a fourteen-year-old girl just beginning to date is very different from the optimal amount of sexual interest deemed appropriate for a twenty-four-year-old newlywed, a forty-four-year-old mother of two, or an eighty-four-year-old widow. Sometimes life and circumstances are not as straightforward as they may seem. Consider the twenty-four-year-old newlywed who has had no sexual experience prior to marriage compared to a twenty-four-year-old newlywed who is also a new mother. What about an eighty-four-year-old widow who has found a male companion or a forty-four-year-old mother who has finally given birth to twins after years of treatment for infertility? What about a woman whose husband wants sex more than once a day or a woman who is married to a man who wants sex only on special occasions?

The optimal amount of sexual interest is what works for each woman in her own unique situation. How do we know when we have found the amount that is just right, the amount of desire that is . . . well, desirable? Trust yourself. You will know it. It won't be a numeric value but rather a feeling that sex is a positive, self-affirming, and integrated part of your life. You won't feel forced or pressured to have sex. You will feel free to say yes or no depending on your inclination. Sex will be an expression of your feelings and a reflection of the quality of your relationship. You will feel good about sex before, during, and after. Whether to have sex will be negotiable, flexible, and will fluctuate depending on other life circumstances. You won't be walking on eggshells around your partner or avoiding intimacy with him. You will feel good in your own skin. So think about sex in the context of your life and not in terms of what the surveys or experts say is normal or ideal.

Putting Sex in Context

We should not be surprised that women's sexual behavior is more reflective of their partner's desire than their own. Many women began their sexual lives this way, having sex because their boyfriend wanted them to. It is rare to hear of a young woman wanting to engage in more extensive sexual activity than her boyfriend wants.[3] Indeed, when we were girls, most of us got the message that our sexual desire was not as strong, as robust, or as urgent as boys' desire. In fact, we were told, implicitly or explicitly, that we were responsible for regulating the desires of the boys who would be taking us on dates, driving us in cars, and escorting us to important functions. As girls, and later as women, we have had to incorporate a variety of factors, beyond physical lust, into our sexual decision making. Most women have had the experience of being responsible for the birth control, use of the condom (to protect us and our partners from sexually transmitted diseases), and regulating when in the relationship intercourse could occur. Instead of recognizing the wisdom and the sensitivity that we must have gained from our experiences, we find ourselves being held up to suspicion when we don't want sex: suspicion of being hormonally imbalanced, overcontrolling, critical, duplicitous, or just plain not sexy.

Women need a reason to have sex, beyond simply satisfying a physical urge that may no longer exist. A woman's sexual feelings evolve over the years and become more finely tuned to the relational and emotional aspects of her life. We learn, as we go through life, what holds the promise of physical pleasure and what does not. We also learn what holds the promise of emotional fulfillment and what does not. Our sexual feelings become informed by our experience. Instead of trying to override our disinterest in sex, we need to listen to what our bodies and our brains are telling us. When our sexual desire goes, it is telling us that something is wrong.

The Roots of Desire

We need to move beyond a simple "drive" model of sex, where sexual desire is assumed to be a natural and automatic reaction to deprivation, much in the same way that hunger and thirst are viewed. A simple drive model in no way encompasses the emotional complexity of sexual relationships. If we assume instead that sexual desire is not automatic but must be elicited, then we can stop blaming women and concentrate instead on what will produce passion.

In adolescence, everything about sex is new and exciting. Our desire for sex can be driven by novelty, by the illicit nature of the activity, or by the thrill and anticipation of pleasure and of making a connection with a new and desirable partner. As we mature, as our relationships progress, and as we have more sexual experiences, the things that once drove our desire will no longer do so. Familiarity may not breed contempt, but it may breed complacency. The important fact is that we can't continue to rely on the same triggers for desire we had as teenagers or as new lovers whatever our age.

Most women come to find that their desire is sparked or inhibited by the interactions they have with their partner. In surveys, many women report that the goal or the objective of sex is to feel close to their partner, and they recognize that feeling close and being close would cause them to feel like having sex.[4] Most men recognize the importance of relationship factors for women's sexual desire, but in one study almost one-quarter of the men interviewed said that they didn't have a clue as to how to inspire passion in their partner. As one man responded, "If I knew the answer to that, I would have an extremely happy relationship."[5]

Women need to know what it is that creates or contributes to their desire for sex. Since this will change over the course of their lifetime—what inspires passion at twenty is different from what interests us at fifty—women need to be able to communicate their knowledge to their partners. We can be sexual throughout our lives, but our sexuality needs to keep pace with the changes we are going through. If we remain aware and in tune with the changes in our lives, we can adapt our sexuality accordingly. The following case provides an abbreviated example of the difficulties that can arise from a failure to evolve.

Me Tarzan, You Jane

Early in my career as a sex therapist, I was consulted by a couple in their late fifties—I'll call them Janet and Todd. It was the second marriage for both. Both had been in very unhappy and sexually un- fulfilling first marriages. Todd had believed he was impotent, but with Janet he found that he was not. Janet never knew that sex could be something exciting for her. Initially she felt tremendously desired and desirable when she was with Todd. She experienced her first orgasm with him. On the surface it appeared that they had a very satisfying sex life. At first they had sex almost every day. They be- longed to a naturist group and vacationed every year at some exotic spot where they could enjoy nudity. But shortly after their marriage, Janet lost her sexual desire. The couple tried almost compulsively to restore the passion they once had. The problem was that their pattern of lovemaking had not changed since they first had sex, but their lives had. They had married and now lived together. It was no longer exciting to see each other the way it had been when they were dat- ing; there was no more anticipation of a romantic evening every time they saw each other. By the time they came to see me, both Janet and Todd could recount in minute detail when, where, and how they would have sex. It was extremely predictable. Janet was afraid not to have sex—she did not want to have a repeat of her first sex- less marriage—so every time her husband initiated sex upon going to bed, Janet acquiesced. Todd was desperately seeking assurance that his wife still desired him, but his anxiety was mounting and his erection problems were returning. The more anxious he became, the more doggedly he stuck to what had worked in the past. Janet wanted to be swept off her feet again. She wanted to be Jane to his Tarzan.[6] Neither Janet nor Todd knew how to have a passionate relationship within a marriage. Once they were able to acknowledge their anxiety and their mutual naïveté, they became more creative lovers. They also stopped having sex every day but were very happy with sex once a week, or sometimes twice, depending on their mood. They realized that even Tarzan and Jane's relationship would have had to change once they left the jungle.

The Desire-Arousal Feedback Loop

Sexual desire is not something that you feel only prior to sex. It is your wish, your motivation, and your physical urge to engage in sex that hopefully precedes and continues throughout a sexual encounter. Sexual desire and sexual arousal are not synonymous. Sexual arousal refers to the physical and psychological sensations that result from sexual stimulation. While the things that turn one person on do not necessarily excite someone else, caresses, passionate kisses, sexually explicit thoughts, and erotic movies are examples of things that can elicit sexual arousal. Like arousal, desire also has a physical component to it. We often feel in our bodies the longing or wish for sex in the same way that we also physically experience emotions such as love, sorrow, and anxiety.

What prompts sexual desire and what results in sexual arousal are often the same when we are young or when we are in a new relationship. The mere thought of our new lover can produce sexual desire *and* get us turned on. Curiosity, sexual arousal, and sexual desire feed off one another. So when we are young or when sex is novel and even somewhat illicit, our sexual interest is accompanied by the first stirrings of arousal, which drives our interest and fans the flames of desire. However, this model does not work well as our relationships mature. After the novelty or the illicit nature of sexual activity wears off, sexual arousal is not so easily generated. The thought of our lover may still bring a smile but no longer arouses us. It is then we require more explicit sexual stimulation, often involving actual physical contact to get excited. And herein lies the conundrum: How do we recognize or feel desire in the absence of arousal? What will inspire us to seek out sexual contact in order to become aroused?

A good relationship often provides the motivation to be sexual, because we are already feeling close to our partner. We may then initiate or respond to intimate touches that are likely to arouse us. Desire leads us to sexual arousal, which in turn increases our sexual desire. This is what I refer to as the desire-arousal feedback loop.

Many women erroneously believe that they lack desire because they do not feel physically turned on prior to sexual activity. While the thought or idea of having sex might have turned us on at one time (and may still do so occasionally), it is a mistake to rely solely on physical stirrings of interest to gauge desire for sex. Why? Because we may not have spontaneous physical urges to have sex as often as we once did or even at all. And as we age, and our relationships age, the idea of sex is less likely to spark a bodily reaction. The physical sensations that are referred to as feeling "horny" or "randy"; the tingling in the genitals; the flushed, warm sensation; the almost imperceptible rise in heart rate and quickening of breath are all in fact signs that we are already sexually aroused. Over time we need to be seduced, touched, or caressed before these feelings occur. Simply put, over time we will increasingly rely on sexual contact to become sexually aroused. Susan's story illustrates a positive relationship between sexual desire and arousal, but it is one in which arousal precedes desire, instead of the other way around.

> Susan felt that she did not have much desire for sex—that is, until her boyfriend approached her. Once he touched her, not in a directly sexual manner but with a romantic, sensual caress, she felt that sex was something she definitely wanted. Susan's feelings were a combination of arousal and desire, and her lovemaking was passionate. The more turned on she was, the more interested she felt. Usually somewhat reserved, Susan was open to and also initiated a variety of sexual activities and sexual play once her boyfriend got the ball rolling. Her boyfriend found her a creative and sensual lover but was perplexed by the fact that she never approached him for sex. At his urging, Susan consulted her gynecologist about her low sexual desire. Her gynecologist referred Susan and her boyfriend to therapy.

Openness to more sexual activity and stimulation during sex is part of sexual desire. Because sexual desire during sex creates and therefore coincides with increasing levels of sexual arousal, it is hard to distinguish the two. But if you think, as Susan did, that you have a desire problem, you may want to examine whether you feel desire once you become aroused. If you do, you can look at the problem differently.

You may understand that you need to be aroused before you experience desire. But you may also want to consider what is going on in your life and in your relationship that does not motivate you to initiate sex. If you don't experience desire during sex itself, you will need to consider whether your initial lack of desire is preventing the desire-arousal feedback loop from working. This was the case for Anna.

> Anna felt no desire to have sex with her husband. When she did have sex with him, she directed all her energies toward pleasing him, touching him, and bringing him to orgasm. She did not want her husband to touch her, and when he did, she would complain of feeling too ticklish, or self-conscious, or irritated. Since Anna did not feel the desire for sex, she was not open to sexual stimulation. Her husband's touch, which once felt very arousing, now resulted in annoyance. Since she limited what she would permit her husband to do, she left little room for the chance that she would become aroused or enjoy the sexual activity. She also left little room for the chance that she would welcome or look forward to a sexual encounter in the future. Outside the bedroom Anna avoided intimate contact with her husband for fear it would lead to sex. Without any physical affection or romantic gestures, sex was always out of context in her marriage.

Past Lives and Loves

Throughout our lives we receive messages from our families, our communities, and our lovers about sex, desire, and intimacy. Sometimes, when we hit a rough, stormy, or stressful patch in our lives, we revert back to what we know best, what we did (or what our mothers did) in the past. If we pay attention, we will know why old patterns are being revived and what direction to take in the future. Knowing what messages you received about sexuality from your parents and from your past experiences may help you understand the situation you are in now and the reaction you are having to it. Brenda and

Margaret, whose stories are told below, had very different reactions to their low sexual desire, reflecting the different attitudes and values they had developed about sex.

Brenda was raised in a loving and sexually permissive family. Her parents had a very good relationship and were openly affectionate with each other and their children. Brenda had always enjoyed her sexuality. She was a very caring person and thought of herself as a giving and generous lover. She placed a high value on sex when it occurred in the context of a loving relationship. When she found herself, after fifteen years of marriage, with no sexual interest for her husband, Brenda was distraught. From the time she was a teenager, her sexual and love interests had always gone together. Now she feared that her loss of interest in her husband meant that she no longer loved him. This thought depressed her tremendously. In therapy Brenda revealed that the stress brought about by her husband's promotion had rendered him irritable and impatient at home. She came to realize that he was no longer behaving as though he loved her, and this caused her to withdraw and lose sexual interest. Her disinterest was a healthy reaction to an unhealthy situation.

Margaret never missed her sexual desire. She always thought she had a low sex drive; in fact, she thought most women did. Margaret's sexual relationship with her husband was mutually satisfying for a time. However, after the birth of their first child, Margaret's husband complained that she never initiated sex and often looked for an excuse not to make love with him. Sex became rather perfunctory, with Margaret often encouraging her husband to "hurry up and finish," assuring him that she was "fine" and had no need of sexual stimulation. Margaret was rather perplexed by her husband's frustration. After all, she often acquiesced when he wanted sex, and she was careful to ensure that they made love at least once a week. She did not understand why sex was not satisfying for him, as he always ejaculated. Margaret came from a traditional Irish Catholic family. Her mother was devoted to her children and constantly sacrificed for them. Sex was never discussed in the family, and Margaret had believed that it was a rather dirty and shameful activity, certainly nothing that a mother should enjoy. When Margaret became a mother herself, many of her dormant beliefs about how she should behave became activated. Her pattern of self-sacrifice extended even to her sexual relationship. Margaret came to therapy because her husband wanted her to.

Putting It All Together

Sexual desire in women is complex and requires our thoughts, our emotions, and our bodies to work in sync. We have to think about sex; specifically, we have to think that sex is right for us. There is no place for desire in coercive sex. Whether it is our first time or our thousandth time, our sexual activity has to be consistent with our personal values and beliefs in order for us to feel desire. We also have to be motivated to engage in sex, which usually means that we have to believe that there is something in it for us (pleasure, pregnancy, and intimacy are some strong incentives). And we have to feel some beginning sexual sensations or at least have faith that our bodies will respond. We have to find our partner desirable, and our relationship has to be supportive enough so that we can feel comfortable having sexual feelings. In order to act on our sexual desire, we have to have the confidence to initiate and respond to sexual overtures. Communication within the relationship has to be clear enough so that sexual invitations, once sent, are received and correctly perceived. Actually, when you think about it, it is almost a miracle that sex occurs at all.

By answering the following questions, you can begin to put your sexual desire into a context—that of your unique life circumstance. Understanding what excites and inhibits your sexual passion and your sexual behavior is vitally important. The remainder of the book will help you further define the problem and guide you to a solution.

• In what situations, if any, do I feel sexual desire? You may feel desire in the middle of lovemaking, you may feel it when you and your partner are apart, or you may feel it when you see an attractive stranger or when you and your partner have been especially close.

• When you experience desire, what comes next? Some women resolve to act on it but never do. Other women feel ashamed and embarrassed because of the circumstances in which they find themselves wanting sex. Some women act on their desire immediately and masturbate if their partner is not available; other women are comforted by the knowledge that this, too, shall pass. Still others initiate sex with a partner.

• Why is your disinterest in sex a problem? Many women are upset because their low desire bothers their partner or they fear a breakup, while others are upset because they miss their sexuality.

• If you do not experience any desire now, and especially if you are not currently in a relationship, look at past situations and experiences to determine under what conditions you've had your interest stirred. This may entail recalling your first crush, or it may require a painful exploration of a divorce or separation.

• Think about the messages that you get about sex, from your parents, siblings, friends, religious community, teachers, the media, boyfriends, men who were your lovers and men who weren't. How have you put all these messages into one coherent statement about your sexuality? For the important people in your life, complete the following sentence: if my (mother, ex-husband, sister . . .) knew about my desire problems, he/she would tell me _____.

Your low sexual desire is a reaction to your life situation. Instead of trying to override your sexual disinterest with hormones, Viagra, or antidepressants, you need to consider what your lack of desire is telling you about your life. Only by addressing the root of the problem can you be assured of creating long-lasting change.

2

Could the Trouble Be Physical?

The omnipresent process of sex, as it is woven into the whole texture of our man's or woman's body, is the pattern of all the process of our life.

HAVELOCK ELLIS

We are physical beings, and a healthy sexual desire presupposes a healthy body. For most women good sex occurs when their minds and bodies are working well and in harmony. It is important to remember that low sexual desire is not a disease in and of itself, just as falling out of love with your partner or losing interest in your work is not considered a disease. In fact, the majority of cases of low sexual desire do not have an identified physical cause. On the other hand, there are certain physical problems that can directly cause a reduction in sexual desire. Emotional factors and stress can also affect you physically and thus affect your libido. So before we turn to what's more likely at the heart of your disastisfaction,

21

let's take a hard look at the role physical conditions might play in your sex life.

Hormones

It is often assumed that a hormonal imbalance is responsible for low sexual desire, although to date there is no evidence showing that there is a difference in the hormone levels of sexually interested and disinterested healthy women. Nevertheless, the usual hormonal suspects are the estrogens, progesterone, prolactin, and the androgens, especially testosterone. (A description of these hormones can be found in Appendix A.)

One of the main reasons that hormonal problems are assumed to underlie low sexual desire is that sexual desire is often disrupted by life events that affect the hormonal balance in the female body. These life events include menopause (surgical or natural), menstrual cycle fluctuations, pregnancy, and the postpartum period. Because women's sexual desire is dependent on so much more than physical stirrings of lust, hormone levels alone are never responsible for our sexual interests and desires. For example, while hormone levels fluctuate during the menstrual cycle, so does our sense of physical and emotional well-being. A woman's sexual activity and interest across the menstrual cycle cannot be predicted by the changes in the level of her hormones. The same is true for pregnancy and the postpartum period. A woman's sexual activity and interest during her pregnancy are more related to how she feels about herself, her pregnancy, her body, and the relationship with her significant other than to what her hormones are doing. After giving birth, many women, especially those who are breast-feeding, do not have high levels of sexual desire for some period of time. While this may be due to elevated prolactin levels or other hormonal changes during the postpartum period, there are equally compelling psychological reasons for reduced sexual interest at this time. The love a woman feels for her new infant, the demands of a newborn, the stress of labor and delivery, and concerns about physical appearance may leave little room for romance in the life of a new mother.

Menopause

Menopause is probably the most maligned hormonal event in the lives of women. Anything that occurs during menopause, especially a decreased interest in sex, is blamed on "the change." Menopause is medically defined as the complete cessation of menses for a duration of one year, although most people think of menopause as the period of time leading up to the end of menstruation when a woman's periods are erratic and infrequent. Perimenopause is actually defined as the process leading up to menopause and involves gradual hormonal changes. Perimenopause can last for ten to fifteen years.

Menopause has been treated as a disease state by many in the medical community rather than as a normal life transition. The collection of symptoms associated with this "disease" is frightening. They include "hot flashes, a stiff and unyielding vagina, wrinkles, shrinking and sagging breasts, aching joints, palpitating organs, frequent urination, itchy skin, osteoporosis, irritability, depression, frigidity, absent-mindedness, loss of memory, and insanity."[1] Recently, all the bad press about menopause has been extended to the perimenopausal phase as well, with women being told that they can expect insomnia, weight gain, memory loss, hot flashes, aching joints, and loss of libido beginning in their thirties.

As a woman ages and passes through the perimenopausal and menopausal stages of her life, the level of her sex hormones (especially estrogen, progesterone, and testosterone) decreases. Women vary dramatically in their physical, emotional, and sexual responses to these changes. While this may be due to different hormonal sensitivity, it may also be due to a woman's attitude about her life. And while her attitude may help determine a woman's response to menopause, her physical response to menopausal changes may also determine her attitude. Naomi and Gail had very different reactions to menopause.

Naomi and David had been married only two years, having met at a group for widows and widowers. Naomi was in her late fifties, and David was sixty-six. Although sex had been pleasant and enjoyable prior to marriage, Naomi was now experiencing pain with intercourse. She was using an estrogen ring to alleviate vaginal dryness in addition to the lubricant she and David used when they had intercourse. Naomi said that all her friends complained of the same problems, and none of them were interested in sex either. Even though Naomi was in a relatively new relationship and even though she loved her husband, she assumed that menopause signaled the end of her sexual pleasure. "Menopause is hard on me," she said, "but it's hard on all the women in my family." Naomi believed that having sex was still her marital duty, but she was fully prepared for the fact that only her husband would enjoy it.

Gail and Dan had been married for thirty-seven years and had four grown children. Dan was a journalist and had traveled a fair bit for his work. Gail had stayed home and raised the children. When the last of their children moved out of the family home and Dan took an editorial job that kept him in one location, Gail was excited. She felt that there was finally going to be time and energy for her. Gail joined a women's hiking group and took up kayaking. She also looked forward to having better sex with her husband and was very disappointed when the perfunctory sex she had attributed to his job stress and lack of time continued. She told Dan that she was not willing to settle and wanted sex to be more fulfilling for her. At fifty-nine Gail was enjoying midlife and the freedom it brought her. She was very motivated to have a good sexual relationship and in fact felt entitled to it.

Dr. Christiane Northrup's bestselling book *The Wisdom of Menopause* has done much to correct the negative impression many North American women have regarding the cessation of their menstrual cycles. Dr. Northrup argues that the passage into menopause and beyond signals a passage into wisdom and a time of greater awareness of oneself and one's own needs and wants. She makes the case that even though hormone levels may be fluctuating in preparation for menopause, it is those women whose lives are out of balance who will suffer the most from these changes. The hormonal swings will bring a woman's buried distress to the surface. She directs women to pay attention to the messages they receive during menopause or during the premenstrual phase of their cycle in order to more fully appreciate what is out of balance. A recent review of the literature on menopause and sexuality[2] has also debunked the myth that menopause signals not just the cessation of the menses but also the cessation of sex. It was a woman's life situation and how she viewed her sexuality, not her menopausal status, that was the important factor in determining her desire to have sex with her partner. As Dr. Northrup states, "A woman with a strong current of life force, who is in love with her life, can continue to have a strong libido regardless of what her hormones are doing."[3] The reverse is also true. A woman with adequate hormones and an unhappy life or relationship will not have a strong sex drive.

Hysterectomy and Oophorectomy

The symptoms of surgically induced menopause following removal of the ovaries will be more severe than if the menopause is "natural." This makes sense, because the rest of your body (not to mention your mind) has little or no time to adapt to the change. Loss of the uterus subsequent to a hysterectomy will negatively affect the sexual experience of those women who enjoyed uterine contractions during orgasm, but it will not necessarily diminish sexual desire if the ovaries are left intact. When the ovaries are removed, there is a significant decrease in estrogen and testosterone, which can result in a variety of sexual problems, including vaginal dryness and loss of desire. In these cases some form of hormone therapy is always recommended.

Not all women who undergo a hysterectomy will have sexual problems. Many women report better sex after the surgery due to the alleviation of their painful symptoms. Research also supports the fact that the more informed you are about what is surgically involved and what the sexual and other side effects may be, the better the post-surgical adjustment.[4] Of course there are also psychological issues involved in any surgery on one's reproductive organs. Some women may feel that they are less feminine, they may need to grieve for their lost reproductive potential, or they may be frightened of injury to the affected area during sex.

Aging

There are a number of life changes that occur at the same time most women are undergoing "the change" that can also account for a decrease in sexual desire. For some women it may be that their children are leaving home, their husband is aging and is experiencing sexual problems of his own, or the woman's career may be either taking off or suffering from the lack of investment over time. Many women at midlife and beyond have lost their partner, due to death or divorce. Health problems associated with aging may also interfere with an active sex life. Either partner may experience decreased energy, strength, and flexibility or may have a serious physical ailment such as heart disease, cancer, or diabetes that interferes with sexual activity and the desire for such activity. If the illness itself does not affect sexuality, it is possible that the medications one takes for it will. A later section in this chapter highlights some of the sexual side effects of many frequently prescribed medications.

Despite all the things that could go wrong with sex as people age, the truth is that for many women sex gets better. The emotional intimacy that comes with good long-term relationships enhances sexual intimacy (of course, it won't resolve itself if intimacy is a troubling issue for you). Many women feel freed from the tyranny of having to aspire to the ideal of beauty, as being older they are no longer eligible for this classification. Postmenopausal women may be experiencing liberation from cumbersome methods of birth control, they may be reveling in the freedom their children's departure provides them, and they may be experiencing a renewed love life, either with a new partner or from renewed interest in a long-term partner. The National Council on Aging[5] conducted a survey of Americans over the age of sixty. The results showed that many older Americans continued to be sexually active and enthusiastic. More than two-thirds of the sexually active women reported that sex was at least as emotionally satisfying as it was in their forties, and 62 percent said that sex was at least as physically satisfying, if not more so, as it was when they were in their forties.

Endocrine Disorders

The endocrine system, and the hormones it produces, is intricately involved in many of the body's functions and is essential to our sense of well-being and our sexuality. The adrenals, which sit atop the kidneys, are the main endocrine glands. They provide vital hormonal support to many of the body's organs and are responsible for producing hormones that help the body respond to the demands of daily life. Overworked adrenal glands can result in low sexual desire. If your adrenals are depleted, you will find that you awake tired and groggy in the morning. You may rely on caffeine and sugar to get through the day, especially in the late morning or afternoon. You may have difficulty falling asleep at night, despite the fact that you are exhausted. Your sex drive will likely be nonexistent. Common causes for adrenal dysfunction include emotional, environmental, and physical stress. Two key hormones produced by the adrenals are cortisol and DHEA. Cortisol enhances your body's natural resistance and endurance. In excess it suppresses the sex hormones and can lead to osteoporosis. DHEA mediates many of the unfavorable effects of excessive cortisol. It is a precursor for testosterone and improves energy, vitality, and mental clarity and helps the body recover from acute stress. When your adrenals are depleted, your cortisol and DHEA levels are out of balance. Adrenal functioning can be restored by diet and lifestyle change, which will necessarily involve addressing the stressors in your life.

Thyroid problems, especially hypothyroidism, can cause low sexual desire. The thyroid is a butterfly-shaped gland located in the lower front of the neck. It produces and releases thyroid hormone (the main one being thyroxine) that regulates body temperature and energy levels and keeps vital organs and various muscles working as they should. Some level of thyroxine appears necessary for the maintenance of sexual desire. In hypothyroidism the thyroid gland does not produce enough thyroid hormone, affecting and slowing down a number of bodily processes. Low levels of thyroid hormone depress androgen levels in the body.[6] Some of the symptoms of hypothyroidism include feeling cold, being easily tired, dry skin, forgetfulness, depression, constipation, heavier and more frequent menstrual cramps, worsened premenstrual symptoms, and low sex drive. Hypothyroidism is more common among women, especially Caucasian and Asian women, and the rate of hypothyroidism goes up during pregnancy, after delivery, and around menopause. The good news is that hypothyroidism can be completely controlled by a daily dose of thyroid hormone replacement. Once the correct dosage has been ascertained, patients experience a significant improvement in symptoms and a return of their sex drive. If you suspect you are hypothyroid, go to your doctor. Hypothyroidism can be detected by a simple blood test.

Another endocrine disorder that affects sexual functioning is diabetes. Male diabetics often experience difficulty getting or maintaining an erection, while women with diabetes report problems with sexual arousal, including lack of lubrication and decreased vaginal or vulvar swelling (because less blood goes to the genitals during sexual stimulation).[7] There is an increase in the incidence of vaginal infections with diabetes, which can complicate matters by causing pain during intercourse. The loss of sexual desire may be secondary to the anticipation of pain, or it may result from the fact that the desire-arousal feedback loop does not work effectively, due to reduced arousal. If you have diabetes, make sure it is under control; otherwise your sexual symptoms will worsen.

Sexually Transmitted Diseases (and Fear of Them)

It is often the psychological reactions, either fear of getting a disease or the shame of having acquired a sexually transmitted disease (STD), that diminish desire. Desire can also be reduced by the pain experienced with some STDs, such as genital herpes or HPV (human papillomavirus) infection, or with the discomfort caused by vaginal or urinary tract infections. A positive test result indicating HIV, the virus believed to cause AIDS, opens the floodgates for a myriad of emotions, including depression, anxiety, and fear. All of these can drastically reduce your sexual desire, especially the fear that you could infect someone you love or the anger you feel at having been infected with an incurable disease. Because the virus attacks the cells of the immune system (whose function is to fight infection and disease), HIV-positive individuals will be susceptible to illnesses that one could normally fend off. These illnesses themselves can cause lower sexual interest. The National AIDS Hotline, (800) 342-AIDS, can provide more information.

For some couples, recurrent STDs disrupt the rhythm of their love-making, and they find it hard to initiate sex after a period of abstinence. Indeed, intense sexual activity interrupted by periods of abstinence (a pattern often seen in long-distance relationships) can actually precipitate vaginal infections. Frequent ejaculations of semen into the vagina over a short time can alter the pH balance of the vagina, inviting infection. When you have sex you don't want, you will notice that your vagina is not well lubricated. The desire-arousal feedback loop is not working; given that you don't have the desire, you will not get as aroused as you otherwise might. The friction of intercourse in a not-well-lubricated vagina is an invitation to irritation and inflammation of the vagina and the urethra. So women with low sexual desire who continue to have sex they don't want or don't enjoy will be prone to more vaginal or urinary-tract infections.

STDs have been around for a long time, and many women have been exposed without experiencing any symptoms. It is not unusual for herpes or genital warts to lie dormant and manifest themselves years after the initial infection. I recently received a call from a very distraught woman. In the sixth month of her pregnancy, she had her first outbreak of herpes. She had been married for eight years. This woman was referred for therapy by her obstetrician because her anxiety and fear about possibly needing to have a cesarean section were extreme. She felt so dirty and ashamed of her condition that she couldn't come in to talk about it. I later heard from her obstetrician that she remained upset and depressed throughout her pregnancy and ultimately had a cesarean section, following an outbreak of herpes.

Instead of asking "Why me?" ask yourself "Why now?" An

immune system depressed by stress, anxiety, lack of sleep, poor diet, or overexertion is less able to fight off infection or maintain a symptom-free status in the presence of an existing HPV or herpes virus. So if you experience an outbreak of herpes or genital warts, or indeed if you get a Pap smear result indicating cervical dysplasia, ask yourself what is out of balance. Ask yourself, "Why am I vulnerable now?" The following case demonstrates the importance of listening to the messages from your body, even if they come in the form of an STD or other kind of infection.

> Celine is the law librarian at a prominent law school. She is an extremely intelligent woman, who, despite being very attractive and athletic looking, lives primarily in her head. Celine was recently divorced from a controlling and demanding husband, and she was disturbed by her recurrent sexual fantasies about one of the law professors at the school where she worked. She was concerned that he, too, was an abusive and controlling sort, and she was upset by her attraction to him. After about six months in therapy, Celine met Jason, a young computer programmer who was rather shy and unassuming. Jason was helping Celine with the installation of computers in the library, and they began a friendship that ultimately became romantic. Although Celine had had genital herpes for over fifteen years, once she began dating Jason, she started to have frequent and severe outbreaks. Celine became so anxious about having an outbreak that she imagined or assumed that she was having one almost constantly. She tried prescription medications, herbal remedies, different underwear, less restrictive clothing, and she changed her soaps and laundry detergent—all to no avail. Celine was convinced that she was a "dirty and corrupting" influence on her more "virtuous" partner. Now that she was not in a relationship where she was being treated badly, her "bad" feelings about herself were being expressed by recurrent outbreaks of herpes. The stress that the herpes caused Celine also caused her to suffer more frequent outbreaks. Once she understood the message inherent in the herpes attacks, she was able to work on improving

her self-esteem. When she felt better about herself, Celine no longer obsessed about infecting or corrupting Jason, and they were able to have a mutually satisfying sexual relationship. Currently herpes is not an issue for Celine, and it has been a year since her last outbreak. Jason remains symptom-free.

Medications

Numerous medications have sexual side effects. Our sexuality is dependent upon so many of our body's systems' working well. Medicating any one of those systems may have an impact on our sexual desire, functioning, and/or pleasure. When a medication lists a possible side effect, it does not mean that everyone will necessarily experience it. However, if your sexual desire is already vulnerable, taking certain medications may tip the balance, and sexual desire problems will become manifest. Some of the more commonly used medications that can result in diminished desire are listed in Appendix B. These include antidepressants, major and minor tranquilizers, sedatives, ulcer medication, and certain blood pressure and heart medications.

The clearest way to know whether the medication you are taking is causing a drop in your sexual desire is to look at the chronology of the problem. If the drop occurred after the medication began taking effect, then it is likely that the medication is at least partly responsible. Ask your doctor if there is another, equally effective medication that you can take that does not have sexual side effects. If not, you have to weigh the benefits and drawbacks of taking the medication. Sometimes you have options, other times you don't. For example, some women do experience reduced sexual desire while taking oral contraceptives. Fortunately, there are other forms of effective birth control that are available. The story is vastly different if you are taking tamoxifen for the treatment of breast cancer—no one would suggest jeopardizing your life in an attempt to increase your sex drive.

Some medications will affect desire because they diminish the sexual pleasure that you would otherwise experience. Again in these cases, ask your doctor if there is another medication that you can take. Consider making lifestyle changes that would be as effective as, and would not come with the sexual side effects of, the medication. Medications that lower blood pressure often have sexual side effects. Proper diet and exercise can also lower blood pressure and will actually enhance sexual pleasure. So while you may need to be on medication for a time, you can also make the lifestyle changes that would allow you to reduce or discontinue the drugs. Once the medication is out of your system, the sexual side effects should disappear as well.

Antidepressants

It may be difficult to know whether the antidepressant you are taking is having an effect on your sexual desire. While loss of sexual desire is a typical side effect of many antidepressants, it is also a symptom of depression. If you notice that the other symptoms of depression are showing improvement, then it is worth considering whether your desire is not returning because of a medication side effect. If switching antidepressants or reducing the dose is not appropriate for you, then doing some of the exercises outlined in the later chapters of this book will help. Another consideration is adding exercise to your treatment plan for depression. Regular exercise has antidepressant effects and may allow you to reduce or discontinue your medication. If you are depressed and are not in therapy, you should be. If your lack of sexual interest is creating real problems in your life and in your relationships, then by taking antidepressants you may be promoting conditions that contribute to depression. It is possible that with therapy the need for medication will lessen and you can reduce or discontinue the medication sooner than you otherwise might. Therapy and exercise should be part of your comprehensive treatment for depression.

Some antidepressants make it more difficult for men and women to reach orgasm. This very common side effect can also affect desire for sex. If your antidepressant interferes with your sexual pleasure, you may need to make some changes in your sexual behavior. You may need to take more time when you have sex or use a vibrator to enhance the stimulation needed for orgasm. If switching, reducing, or stopping the medication are not options, you may need to concentrate on the sexual pleasure you *do* experience and understand that your orgasms will return when you discontinue the medication.

Oral Contraceptives

Some of the birth control options available to women do result in diminished sexual desire, although the hormonal effects are often offset by the freedom from worrying about pregnancy. There are reports that some women taking birth control pills, especially those that are progestin dominant (such as Ortho 7/7/7, Cyclen, and Tricyclen), complain of a decrease in sexual desire as well as vaginal dryness.[8] Research has failed to demonstrate any significant differences in the sexual side effects of different contraceptive formulations. Norplant and Depo-Provera are long-term contraceptives that are made from synthetic progestins. Although there is a rather shocking lack of research on these newer contraceptive methods, anecdotal reports indicate that diminished desire may also be associated with their use. Depo-Provera, a progestin-based contraceptive, is actually used to curb sexual desire in convicted sex offenders!

Fertility Treatment

Many women feel betrayed by their bodies when they want to get pregnant and find they cannot. Their inability to conceive or carry a pregnancy to term is perceived as an assault not only on their capabilities as women but on their sense of themselves as sexual beings. Women who are undergoing treatment for fertility problems usually take hormones to regulate their menstrual cycles, release eggs from the ovaries, and prepare the uterus for implantation of a fertilized egg. Many of these hormonal preparations have an effect on mood and list "emotional irritability" among their common side effects. However, because these medications may further reduce your sense of physical and emotional well-being, and because the necessity of taking them may further damage your sense of competence, it is only logical that your sexual desire will suffer as well. The only drug that specifically lists decreased libido as a side effect is gonadotropin releasing hormone (GnRH), with brand names such as Lupron, Lupron Depot, goserelin, naferelin, Synarel, and Zoladex. These medications are also prescribed for women with endometriosis, uterine fibroids, severe premenstrual syndrome (PMS), and heavy menstrual bleeding.

Sexual desire is not necessary for reproduction, and many of the reproductive technologies either require sex on a schedule or do not require sex at all (as with in vitro fertilization). It is more common than not for women and their partners to experience persistent problems with sexual desire when undergoing fertility treatments. This appears to be a consequence of ignoring or bypassing desire for an extended period of time rather than the result of any lasting physical effects of the fertility drugs. Many couples also have sexual desire problems when they begin treatment for infertility. Unsuccessful attempts to get pregnant tend to associate sex with failure rather than pleasure. So while the physical effects of fertility treatment will disappear once the hormones are out of your system, the psychological effects may linger. Many couples report that it takes a year or more to get their sex lives back on track.

Using Medication to Increase Desire

The centuries-old race to find a drug that will increase sexual desire continues with renewed vigor. Raw oysters, ground rhinoceros horn, alcohol, and various herbs have all been touted as aphrodisiacs at one time or another. The pharmaceutical industry is hoping to cash in by discovering a "cure" for low sexual desire that actually works. However, as long as relationship or other psychological issues are interfering with sexual desire, there will be no improvement from medication alone. Still, several drugs are currently being tested and promoted for their potential to increase sexual desire in women.

Testosterone

Although testosterone is being promoted as the hormone of desire, it is not a sexual panacea. In cases where women's testosterone levels have been reduced (by medication, by surgical removal of the ovaries, or by estrogen therapy for menopausal symptoms), there is evidence that giving women testosterone will reverse any sexual side effects they were suffering, especially low sexual desire. However, women with no hormonal deficit do not benefit from additional testosterone. In cases where low desire is accompanied by life stress, relationship problems, physical illness, or prior sexual problems, testosterone therapy is unlikely to have a positive impact.[9]

Testosterone will purportedly boost our energy, give us more lean body mass, and increase our libido. Of course, so will time spent exercising, eating healthy foods, and being in positive relationships. The problem is that it takes more time and effort to have a healthy lifestyle than it does to pop a pill. Still, given the fact that the short-term benefits of any hormone replacement therapy need to be weighed against the long-term risks, it appears ill advised to use a hormonal preparation in the absence of a diagnosed hormonal deficit.

DHEA

Many women have tried to boost their sexual desire by taking over-the-counter preparations of DHEA, a substance that the body converts to testosterone and then to estrogen. There are still not enough studies on this product to determine its risks and benefits.

Viagra

Despite the success of Viagra in treating erection problems in men, it has not been found to be effective for improving sexual satisfaction in women. Testing is still under way to see if Viagra can be helpful to women who have a diagnosed medical problem that interferes with the blood supply to the genitals during sexual excitation. Viagra does not have an impact on sexual desire in men or women, except indirectly (by improving erections in men with physical problems). Taking Viagra will not increase your sexual desire.

Wellbutrin (Bupropion Hydrochloride)

This antidepressant has been found to have mild stimulating effects. It is being tested to determine whether it will increase sexual desire in women. Currently it is often added to the drug regimen of depressed patients to counteract the sexual side effects of the antidepressants they are taking.

Recreational Drugs

Many women have tried to get in the mood by drinking alcohol or smoking marijuana. If getting in the mood requires these or other recreational drugs, perhaps getting in the mood is not worth it. Using drugs to override your own judgment is never a good idea. Chronic use of alcohol, cocaine, and narcotics can result in permanent damage to your sexual health, including your desire.

Your Body Is Trying to Tell You Something

Low sexual desire is not a disease. It is the understandable result of an imbalance in your life. The imbalance can be in your relationship, your life circumstances, or your body. Even if your low desire has roots in an illness or is a side effect of necessary medication, the exercises and recommendations made in this book can be relevant and useful. Your psychological health and happiness will often determine whether you succumb to an infection, are disturbed by natural changes in your body (menstrual cycle fluctuations, menopause, pregnancy), or experience unwanted side effects of the medications you are taking. Our bodies are amazing in their complexity, and we need to respect the natural tendency to health that is inherent in them. Often our bodies will manifest the symptoms of distress if we fail to notice and address problems. They may continue to be symptomatic if we don't adequately deal with the real issues responsible for our unhappiness, as Wendy and Robert's story illustrates.

Robert felt entitled to sex when he wanted it, and his wife, Wendy, believed that it was her responsibility to satisfy him. Inevitably after they had sex, Wendy would experience irritation and burning in her vagina and urethra. In part this was Wendy's way of expressing her hurt as a result of her husband's insensitivity. It was also a way she had of saying no to sex. Wendy experienced recurrent urinary tract infections followed by yeast infections brought about by the antibiotics she had to take. All of this perpetuated a cycle of frequent but obligatory sex alternating with long periods of abstinence. Wendy finally listened to the message that her body was trying to give her. She told Robert she was "pissed off," and she began refusing to have sex she didn't want. They went to therapy, during which time Wendy had sex with Robert only when she really felt like it. She did not have a recurrence of the urinary tract infections. The couple ultimately divorced, and Wendy is now happily remarried. Despite the fact that her new husband works for a moving company and is often on the road for long periods of time, the pattern of frequent (but enjoyable) sex separated by periods of no sex has not resulted in any vaginal or urinary tract infections.

Our sexuality is dependent upon our emotional and physical well-being. When one aspect of our life is out of balance, it will upset other aspects as well. While it is important to medically address physical symptoms, it is also important to determine what, if any, are the emotional underpinnings of the problem. Wendy's frequent urinary tract infections, while physically real, were also a reaction to her unhappy sexual relationship.

3

Why Don't I Feel the Way I Used to Feel?

*Natural sex, like a natural brassiere,
is a contradiction in terms.*

LEONORE TIEFER

The model of love and sexual desire that comes from television, movies, books, and songs gives us the message that true love is all-consuming and obsessive. The sexual passion that is inspired by such love is powerful and overwhelming. It supersedes our best judgment and often leads us astray. In great literature we see this message repeated over and again. From the brooding Heathcliff in *Wuthering Heights* to Anna Karenina to the English Patient in Michael Ondaatje's novel of the same name, men and women love passionately, obsessively, and recklessly. Such love rarely ends well. We close the pages or leave the movie theater with tears in our eyes but also with a resolve in our hearts that this kind of love is the love for us.

Such passion is always short-lived. It throws us off balance, and we can stay in this state of disequilibrium for only so long. We strive for balance in our lives. For most women, at some point in their lives, passion is in the pursuit of love and a stable, long-term, harmonious relationship. Even the women in HBO's hit series *Sex and the City* are looking for lasting love while they enjoy or struggle through one affair after another. So while we may know that this heady, intoxicating feeling will not last forever, most of us want some romance, some adventure, and a lot of love in our lives. When we reach the point of feeling none of the above, we must take heed that our lives are again out of balance. This time, however, the imbalance is not exciting or intoxicating. On the contrary, it is a more subtle malaise, a tedium that can be tolerated or endured for quite some time.

Our sexual feelings provide us with important information about the nature and quality of our life and our relationships. When our sexual desire disappears, we should not attribute this to the inevitable result of being in a long-term relationship. It is a message that something in our life is out of balance; something is wrong. If we believe that wild, reckless passion is love, then when it is gone we will believe that we have fallen out of love. Some people constantly seek this passion and consequently rarely end up in long-term, monogamous relationships. They may marry but soon get divorced, or they may find themselves in one affair after another. This does not mean people should stay in a relationship no matter how dull and boring it is. Some relationships may not withstand the test of time and are better short-lived. Love, romance, passion, and excitement are not experienced in the same way over the course of a forty-year marriage as they are in obsessive love affairs. Sexual disinterest is often the canary in the coal mine, the early warning signal that there is a problem. Whether the relationship will stand the test of time will depend on many other factors (love, commitment, children, and so on).

Balance

The message here is that balance is the key. Obsessive love signals that there is something missing in our own life, something we're trying to find in someone else. At the extreme are women who become groupies to rock stars or athletes, who want to achieve some status by borrowing it from another. Many women in the throes of obsessive love feel that they will die without their beloved. When we experience the opposite and have no passionate feelings for our partner, it is a signal to us as well that something is missing, something is not right, something is out of balance.

Ask yourself the following questions. Your answers will allow you to see where the source of your disinterest lies, where the imbalance exists.

Answer true or false in response to the following statements:

1. Though I rarely initiate sex, I enjoy it when it happens and wonder why I don't have sex more often. _____

2. Most often I have sex just to please my partner. It is not for my own pleasure. _____

3. Sex is not very exciting for me. I don't see what all the fuss is about. _____

4. I used to be very interested in sex, but lately that has changed. _____

5. The men I date are not interested in having a long-term relationship with me. (If you are not in a committed relationship, answer from past experience.) _____

6. My partner does not really turn me on sexually. He is not a very good lover. _____

7. I often fake orgasm or enjoyment during sex. _____

8. I am very aware of when we have sex, and I try to make sure that we have sex on a routine basis. _____

9. I am worried that my partner will leave me if he doesn't get enough sex. _____

10. I spend a great deal of time worrying about how I look. _____

11. I don't believe that my partner is sexually attracted to me. _____

12. It's my pattern to lose interest in sex once the initial thrill of the relationship is over. _____

13. Other people would never think of me as sexy. _____

14. I find myself fantasizing about other people. I am sexually attracted to men (or women) other than my partner. _____

15. I initiate sex to avoid arguments with my partner. _____

16. There is not enough time to have sex on a regular basis. _____

17. My partner is too needy sexually. _____

18. I often find myself resentful of my partner's sexual needs. _____

19. My partner often makes sex go on and on. If it could take less time and energy, there might be more of a place for it in my life. _____

20. At some point in my life, I have been made to do sexual things I didn't want to do or didn't understand. _____

21. I often get anxious or panicked during sex. _____

22. I really believe I need to get out of this relationship. _____

23. Lust is a dangerous thing. _____

24. My partner has cheated on me. _____

25. I have cheated on someone I was or am involved with. _____

A woman's sexual disinterest usually results when there is an imbalance in one or more areas of her life and her significant relationship. The eight areas of most concern are:

1. Control and power
2. Intimacy
3. Sexual self-esteem
4. Stress
5. Unresolved anger
6. Sexual dysfunction
7. Trauma
8. Abuse

What follows is a description of these imbalances and their impact on sexual interest. Your answers to the preceding questions should help you to pinpoint which ones are descriptive of your unique situation. Remember, disequilibrium can occur in more than one area, and problems in one aspect of your life may beget problems in others.

Control and Power

You may have answered true to some or all of these questions: 2, 4, 7, 8, 9, 15, and 18.

Many women relinquish their independence when they marry or partner, unaware that their independence was the wellspring of their passion. They don't do this consciously. They don't automatically get into the passenger seat of the car because they are intentionally giving up their power. They tell themselves (if they think of it at all) that "he likes to drive, and I don't really care." The woman may keep track of the checkbook, but he makes the investment decisions. His career takes precedence over hers because . . . because it just does. She may believe that his career is more important than hers because he makes more money. It is easy to forget that equal pay for work of equal value is still a goal for the future. As working women, we were supposed to have parity with our husbands. However, as Arlie Hochschild describes in *The Second Shift*,[1] women who work outside the home still do most of the housework and child care. We are still operating under the old rules even though they no longer make sense. All of this is worsened for the woman raised in a family where men were dominant and women submissive. This was Michelle's situation.

Michelle's parents married in their late thirties after a very tumultuous courtship that was marked by frequent separations, including a time when her father was engaged to another woman. Michelle's mother was desperate to get married. She felt that her self-worth was dependent upon it. After the marriage Michelle's mother continued to act as though she were worthless and her husband all-powerful, even though she came to bitterly resent his casual and abusive treatment of her. Michelle's mother had no control of the family's finances, had only a minor say in mundane decisions, and had no say at all in matters of importance. Michelle grew up determined that her life would be different from her mother's. She spent her twenties working as a teacher and traveling all around the world. She eventually got her Ph.D. and was hired to teach at a very prestigious university. She was highly regarded in professional circles. In her late thirties, Michelle married Tony, a man she was passionately in love with. He was a secondary-school teacher who had attended one of her training programs. Several years into the marriage, Michelle realized she was indeed living her mother's life. She found herself resentful of Tony, believing that he was the reason she was not leading the exciting life she had led before her marriage. Indeed, Michelle had begun to act like her mother and to treat her husband as though he were her father. She cooked the foods Tony liked, listened to the music Tony liked (saving her favorite CDs for solo car trips), and soon stopped watching sitcoms because Tony thought they were frivolous. Michelle stopped attending conferences and did her work quietly, so as not to upstage her husband. She did not travel very often because Tony tended to be a homebody. She acted as though she had no power in the relationship, as though she were not as worthwhile as her husband. It is not surprising that she lost her passion.

Women have been led to believe that the only power they possess lies in pleasing other people. Women who direct their energies solely to meeting other people's needs and expectations have lost touch with their own pleasure. While they may engage in sexual activity, all too frequently it is only for the other person's benefit. They never initiate sex because they feel desire. They may initiate sex because they believe that the other person expects it, wants it, or will become angry if sex does not occur. Such was the case with Donna.

Donna was married to a successful businessman. When they were in college together, they had an active and imaginative sex life. Once they decided to marry, Donna dropped out of school to support Michael while he pursued his M.B.A. Although the plan was for Donna to resume school later on, she never did. Once married, Donna lost her desire for sex. Although she still had sex with Michael, he could tell that she was just "going through the motions." Soon they stopped having sex altogether. Donna was desperate to get her sexual desire back, because she knew it would make Michael happy. Donna had completely lost touch with herself and her own passions, sexual and otherwise.

If a sense of personal empowerment feeds desire, then powerlessness drains it. There is an ancient Greek story of a woman, Lysistrata, who, tired of war, led her sister wives in a resistance movement. Unable to get their husbands to listen to their entreaties for peace, they vowed not to "raise their slippers in the air" until the war was ended. In other words, they agreed not to have sex until their husbands let them have a voice in how their lives would be lived. It is unfortunate when the only power one can possess lies in refusal. It is rare, however, for the refusal to be such a conscious manipulation as that orchestrated by Lysistrata. In some relationships women may feel, or they may be told, that they must have sex at their partner's desire and discretion. If saying no is not an option, then yes becomes meaningless. When you believe and act as though your sexual desire is irrelevant, as if it is not important in terms of your decision about whether to have sex, then your desire will fade and disappear. It will have become obsolete.

In order to restore your desire, you will need to restore your sense of personal empowerment. You can accomplish this by doing the exercises in the remainder of the book. These exercises will help you get in touch with lost or neglected sexual feelings and will help you bring your desire back into your sexual decision making and ultimately back into the relationship.

Intimacy

You may have answered true to some or all of the following questions: 4, 5, 12, 14, 17, 18, 24, and 25.

"Why is it that the men I want don't want me, and the ones who want me . . . well, I don't want them?" If this is or was a familiar complaint, making an intimate connection may be difficult for you. Women who have once had a high interest in sex and who lose this interest once they are in a committed relationship are often avoiding intimacy by avoiding sex. They may justify their disinterest in a variety of ways: they may blame their partner's poor sex skills, his lack of romance, his bad temper, his sloppy hygiene, or any number of things. But the bottom line is that they do not address the issues they complain about so that sexual intimacy can occur. In truth, they are not interested in having sex and their complaints justify their lack of desire. Instead of asking, "Why are all the men I'm attracted to not interested in me?" turn the question back on yourself. Ask instead, "Why am I not interested in men who are available and interested in having a relationship with me? What am I afraid of?"

The answer to this question can come from many sources. Look back at the family you were born into. Whether you like it or not, your parents were your first role models for making intimate connections, not only in how they related to one another but in how they related to you. If you did not get the basis for intimacy in your family, it is often difficult to be close and loving in your adult relationships. Thomas Fogarty, a psychiatrist and family therapist, wrote, " Unlike distancing from another person, closeness must be accomplished gracefully." [2] Anna represents a woman who has tried to restore her passion for her husband without resolving her fear of intimacy. In one of her therapy sessions, Anna reported the following dream and her thoughts about it:

> "I am with Kevin, the only other man I've really loved other than my husband. Well, I'm with Kevin, I've found him, tracked him down. He's left his wife or girlfriend to be with me. We are having sex, and it's great. Then he goes out for a loaf of white bread or a beer or something, and he doesn't come back. He's left me. But I know I will find him again, I will track him down, and I will be with him again. It's that feeling that I don't want to wake up from. That I'm addicted to. The pursuit. The manipulation. The twisting yourself into a pretzel for the other person. . . . When I lost my virginity, I read every book I could on sex: *How to Make Love to a Man, How to Make Love to a Woman.* I wanted to have the best technique. It's like someone handed me a weapon. Some reason for men to be with me. I could give them sex. It's just . . . I don't know what to do with them when I have them."

What Anna is describing is not uncommon for women who have low sexual desire. In a committed relationship, sex is a way to express and enjoy intimacy. For many women, their past experiences have led them to view sex primarily as a way to draw someone to them. Sex can also be used as a means to avoid intimacy, a way to give something to the relationship without really revealing one's true self.

Once in a committed relationship, these women complain of sexual boredom, lack of sexual desire, and even an aversion to sex. Like Anna, these women are at a loss in intimate relationships. If they could not maintain a "safe" distance, these women would be highly anxious in their relationships or would avoid relationships altogether. If Anna's story sounds familiar, you might want to ask yourself:

- What is it about intimacy that I want to avoid?
- Is it truly my husband or boyfriend whom I want to avoid, or is it that I don't know how to be intimate?
- Has my partner hurt my feelings, communicated in some way to me that it is not safe to share myself, or did I get that feeling from elsewhere?

Remember that water seeks its own level. If you are currently in a committed relationship, it is likely that your partner is not any more comfortable with intimacy than you are. In other words, the problem is not all yours, although you are the one who is maintaining the distance. If you get closer, your partner may begin to distance. This is why restoring intimacy (sexual and emotional) needs to proceed gradually, so that you both have time to get comfortable with the closeness. Bringing your sexual desire to the relationship is an intimate act, and it makes many women feel anxious and vulnerable. Following the step-by-step approach to restoring sexual desire that is outlined in the remainder of this book will help you gradually and gracefully bring your sexual desire back into the relationship.

Sexual Self-Esteem

You may have answered true to some or all of the following questions: 1, 9, 10, 11, 13, 24, and 25.

Women who don't feel entitled to be objects of desire lack desire themselves. As one woman complained, "I don't want to want what I can't have." Women may be highly capable and confident in many areas of their life, but if they do not believe that they are sexually desirable, they may suffer from a poor sexual self-image or low sexual self-esteem.

Prevailing societal attitudes and cultural myths about beauty and attractiveness contribute greatly to this problem. Many of us are led to believe that the current cultural definition of beauty is also the definition of sexy. We don't make the same mistake when it comes to men. While many attractive men are deemed sexy, many physically unattractive men also fall into the category. The classic example has always been Woody Allen, who, before his fall from grace, was considered one of the sexiest men in America. Take a good look at many male rock stars or athletes who are considered sexy but would not stand a chance in a men's beauty pageant. We find men sexy who make us laugh, who are highly accomplished or extremely intelligent. Why is it not the same for women?

Of course, much of the problem lies in our beliefs about what men want. Men's magazines such as *Playboy,* with its airbrushed centerfolds, contribute to the notions that sexiness is beauty and that men are turned on simply by looking. While this may be true to some extent, unless your boyfriend or husband is a voyeur, he will want some interaction and interest on your part. Older men especially need to be touched, stroked, or caressed in order to get aroused. Despite the messages from commercials, perfect hair, teeth, a flat stomach, and perky breasts may make you good to look at but won't in and of themselves make you a good lover or a sexy woman. Sexy is attitude. It says, "I am open to giving and receiving pleasure." This message may be one that is publicly conveyed, or it may be a private understanding between you and your partner.

Low sexual self-esteem can be chronic or life circumstances can contribute to it. Weight gain (even during or after pregnancy), aging, job loss, divorce, and a partner's infidelity or habitual neglect can all contribute to making a woman feel undesirable. Even if one's partner continues to profess interest, this interest is often perceived as disingenuous or simply self-serving. Women with low sexual self-esteem often think of men's sexual interest as a physical urge unrelated to love or intimacy. Such women often do not feel entitled to express their sexual preferences, and so sex is not as enjoyable as it could be.

Women who don't feel entitled to be desired don't feel desirable. This was the case with Heather.

> Heather spent a lot of time in front of the mirror deciding what to wear. She usually rejected one or two outfits before she finally re-signed herself to the fact that she needed to get dressed and would have to accept the way she looked. Heather felt that she was un-attractive. Cosmetic surgery on her nose as an adolescent had not helped her feel better about herself. Spending a lot of money on clothes did not help, either. Heather's father had fancied himself quite the ladies' man and had commented on how women looked since the earliest time Heather could remember. Heather had grown up placing inordinate value on appearances. Although she was smart and professionally successful, she did not value these accomplishments. Heather was married at a young age, after she discovered she was pregnant. Twenty years later she continued to feel that her husband did not choose to be married to her. Her re-lationship was in serious trouble after years of little or no sexual contact between her husband and herself. While Heather's self-esteem had improved in other areas, she needed to improve her self-esteem in the context of her sexual relationship.

Some women with low sexual self-esteem have recognized their own sexual attractiveness only after having an affair. Unfortunately, this usually signals the end of their marriage. It is essential that the im-provement in sexual self-esteem occur in the context of the relation-ship if the relationship is going to survive.

Low sexual self-esteem may be one part of a larger self-esteem issue, and dealing with it may represent only one aspect of a larger goal to improve one's overall sense of self-worth. Women with low self-esteem act as though they are unimportant. Women with low sex-ual self-esteem act as though they are not sexy, not sexually desirable, and certainly not sexually desirous. Their lives continue to be a self-fulfilling prophecy: "I am not sexy, therefore I am not entitled to de-sire. Sex is a problem in my relationship, therefore I know I am not sexy." If you have low sexual self-esteem, it is important to break this self-defeating cycle. Do the exercises in the following chapters. As you get in touch with your sexual desire and learn how to integrate it into your relationship, you will break the cycle and a new one will take its place: "I feel sexual desire, sex is an important and enjoyable part of my relationship, and therefore I know I am sexy."

Stress

You may have answered true to some or all of the following questions: 1, 4, 16, 17, 18, and 19.

In Carol Ellison's book *Women's Sexualities,*[3] she notes that many women cite stress as the number-one factor that inhibits their sex lives. She surveyed more than twenty-six hundred women and found that the top three concerns they noted were "being too tired to have sex," "being too busy," and "having lower sexual desire than I wanted to have." North Americans now work harder and longer than at any other time in our history. Working twelve hours a day does not lend itself to long hours of romance at night. Women continue to carry the burden of household and child-care responsibilities. This can lead to buried resentments and anger. Indeed, Ellison quotes one of her survey respondents as writing, "I'm too tired to have sex and resentful about housework. I need a full-time maid!"

Stress also contributes to bad behavior overall. Put lab mice into stressful, overcrowded living conditions and they attack one another. Nasty remarks, short tempers, and never having enough time for each other do not bode well for having a physically and emotionally satisfying sexual relationship. Foreplay doesn't just start in the bedroom. It comes from helping to get the kids dressed in the morning, pouring a cup of coffee for your partner, warming the car, asking about her day, listening to her stories. A very old cartoon from the *New Yorker* shows a man on bended knee before a seated woman who exclaims, "Oh, how wonderful that you would do anything for me. Could you start by vacuuming the rug?"

Marriage is more stressful for women than it is for men, or at least it is stressful in a different way. Following a divorce, women speak about a burden being lifted, that burden being their almost constant preoccupation with what their husbands were thinking, feeling, and wanting from them.[4] Often this type of stress leads women to want to distance themselves from their husbands, to get some time alone, or to spend time with girlfriends for whose emotions they do not have to feel responsible. If women agonize about their partner's feelings regarding television shows, recreational activities, dinner menus, and home décor, imagine the stress and pressure to take care of their partner's sexual feelings. This does not mean that a woman acquiesces every time she thinks her boyfriend or husband wants to have sex. It means that her decisions about whether to have sex are always tinged with a concern about her partner's reactions and are not based solely on her own desire. She doesn't want to hurt his feelings, she doesn't want to say no too often, so she may try to avoid the problem altogether by avoiding intimate contact. This also gives her some breathing room from the burdensome responsibility of someone else's happiness and self-esteem. The fallout is that relationships become more distant and strained, and sex becomes a duty, not a pleasure. If sex is on the to-do list, and not part of the rest-and-relaxation program, it will become an activity that is avoided as stresses pile up. Jennifer's story attests to this.

> Jennifer took great pride in her appearance, in her home, and in her work. After the birth of her first child, Jennifer was determined to add "perfect mother" to her list of accomplishments. In order to make more money, her husband, Bill, increased his hours at work. This created more stress for Jennifer. Although she read articles on stress reduction, they did not seem to apply to her life. She couldn't take a long soak in the tub after a hard day's work, and she couldn't afford the time, let alone the money, for massages, manicures, or yoga class. Meditation? Not when shopping lists, doctor's appointments, errands, and a crying baby kept interrupting the flow. Jennifer began to resent any intrusion on her time and energy. She knew that her husband was working hard and bringing in a bigger paycheck. She berated herself for not being more considerate of his feelings, but when he got home from work, she wanted a break from the house and the baby. Jennifer didn't want to have to take care of Bill now, too. She began to resent his sexual advances. Didn't he know she needed to sleep? If she had sex now, and it took twenty

minutes, she could still get six and a half hours' sleep, according to her calculations, but if the baby woke up early or if she wanted to throw a wash in before she went to work . . . Needless to say, Jennifer felt no sexual desire and indeed found her husband's desire inappropriate and insensitive.

If sex has been an obligation, it will be difficult to imagine it's all of a sudden becoming something that you do to rest, relax, and rejuvenate. But this does not have to happen all at once. First you have to have time for rest and relaxation, and this may require making adjustments in your busy life. Not necessarily an easy task. As you follow the steps in this book, reclaiming your desire will help you to feel that time and space for yourself and for you and your partner to enjoy each other are important.

Unresolved Anger

You may have answered true to some or all of questions 4, 6, 14, 17, and 18, and false to 2, 9, and 11.

Unresolved issues in a relationship can lead to buried resentments and seething anger. Anger is such a strong emotion that it will exhaust the hardiest among us. It is also an emotion that creates distance between people. When you are angry with someone, you do not feel like being open and vulnerable to him or her. Anger is also an important signal that something is wrong, usually that someone has transgressed or violated a boundary. While you may be angry that your husband has forgotten to put out the trash again, the source of your anger comes from the message you infer from his forgetfulness: that what you need is unimportant or that you are not being listened to. And not feeling angry about something anymore doesn't always mean that things are settled. Couples who work out issues even with heated arguments are better off than couples who try to be nice all the time but resolve nothing. Underground anger kills passion. This was the problem for Lorna.

Lorna had always been told that she had a bad attitude and a bad temper. When she met and married Tom, everyone commented on how easygoing and nice he was. Lorna and Tom never argued. If Lorna brought up a problem, Tom immediately apologized and accepted blame. However, Tom continued to do pretty much as he pleased without consulting Lorna, and he would apologize profusely if she became upset. On one occasion Tom accepted a new job that required him to travel 50 percent of the time, despite the fact that Lorna was eight months pregnant with their second child. Lorna was furious, and Tom apologized over and over again, but what could he do? He had already resigned and accepted the new position. Lorna remained angry with Tom, even though she had no avenue to express it. Her passion for him diminished to the point that she could not bear to have him touch her. It was only after she recognized the legitimacy of her feelings and demanded real change in the relationship that her desire for Tom returned.

If you believe that there are unresolved issues that block your sexual desire, it is important for you to address them. Your lack of desire is a strong message to you, and it will also be one for your partner. Your partner's interest in improving your sexual relationship may provide the motivation for him to listen to your concerns and address the problems in the relationship. Sex is not a bargaining chip. You don't want to say, "If you take out the trash, I will have sex with you." But you do want to tell your partner that you have anger about some unresolved issues and that this anger kills your sexual desire for him. What you want is discussion and some resolution. You may not always get your way about something, but you should come away from discussions feeling listened to, understood, and appreciated. Your sexual desire should then return.

There are two reasons that it might not. First, sexual problems often take on a life of their own, and you and your partner may find yourselves locked in the routine of sexual avoidance. Second, it is often hard to let go of issues even when they have been discussed and resolved. So even though you know that your partner understands how you feel when he "forgets" to do things around the house, and even though you can see that he is making an effort, you cannot let go of the hurt and anger you once felt, and you do not feel sexually interested. If your sexual desire does not return after the anger has been resolved, then take the step-by-step approach outlined later in the book to reintroduce sex and desire to your relationship. You will want to pay special attention to the sections on communication.

Sexual Dysfunction

You may have answered true to some or all of questions 2, 3, 4, 6, 7, 14, and 18 and false to question 1 if you believe that your partner may have sexual difficulties. If you believe that the problem may be yours, you may have answered true to some or all of questions 2, 3, 7, 13, and 21 and false to question 1.

Sexual problems and the way one deals with them can have a major impact on sexual desire. Sometimes such problems result from anxiety and insecurity about sexual performance. When they do, it is likely that there will also be anxiety and insecurity about addressing these problems. Anxious men and women will often turn to sex manuals for tips on technique. Sometimes helpful, these manuals may give detailed advice on how to stimulate a particular spot but offer only vague generalities regarding how to communicate about sex with your lover. Sometimes just buying the book and saying, "Let's try this," is sufficient, but sometimes it is not. It is not unusual for people who are insecure about their abilities as a lover to buy a book and read it in private, hoping to later astonish their partner with their improved performance. Women, who tend to feel responsible for all sorts of problems in a relationship, may turn to self-help books to find out how to help their partner without his even having to acknowledge the fact that there is an issue. But most often sexual difficulties arise when couples fail to communicate with each other.

Even if the problem is physical, such as erection problems due to diabetes, it's worse when communication is poor. One newly married young woman was so embarrassed by her genital herpes that she avoided her husband altogether when she felt there was a chance of an outbreak. Although her husband was aware of her herpes, she could never bring herself to explain that she needed to abstain from intercourse and oral sex for a good reason. Her husband was perplexed by her avoidance of him at what appeared to be random intervals, and he became anxious and insecure.

It is hard to be enthusiastic about sex if it's not very satisfying. But it is not a particular sexual problem per se that causes desire to wane as much as it is how a couple deals with it. If the person manifesting the problem refuses to do anything about it—including talk about it—the situation appears hopeless. As long as the couple can discuss their situation and look for resolutions, desire usually persists. The following two cases demonstrate the difficulties that can arise from an imbalance in sexual functioning.

Mindy had been disappointed with Calvin's lovemaking for years. No sooner would they start having sex than it would be all over. Calvin suffered from premature ejaculation. Although he would often insist on pleasuring Mindy after he had ejaculated, Mindy felt dissatisfied and frustrated. Everything that Calvin tried in order to maintain better control over the timing of his orgasm inhibited hers (including the anesthetic cream he rubbed on his penis, which then rubbed off on her genitals). Mindy lost interest in sex. It just wasn't a pleasurable experience for her. Although she knew what the cause of her disinterest was, she did not know how to broach the subject to Calvin, nor did she know what could be done about it. Sex became less and less frequent, which made Calvin's problem worse. As the premature ejaculation worsened, Mindy's pleasure decreased even more, and a destructive cycle of avoidance and displeasure was in place.

Beth had never had an orgasm. Still, she wasn't too concerned about it. She valued the emotional closeness and intimacy that sex afforded her. All this changed when she met and married Matthew. Matthew was determined to be the one who rescued Beth, who gave her an orgasm. Never mind that this was not of much interest to Beth. Soon, however, it began to bother her. She felt pressured to have an orgasm to reassure her husband that he was a good lover. Eventually that sense of intimacy and closeness gave way to performance demand and anxiety. Not much longer after that, Beth lost her desire for sex.

Most, if not all, sexual problems can be resolved. Sometimes this will require the services of a sex therapist or a marriage counselor. Sometimes a urologist or a gynecologist can help. But the key to a good sexual relationship is always communication. First there needs to be an acknowledgment that there is a problem and an agreement on what should be done. Then there needs to be ongoing communication regarding the progress you are making. Each partner needs to feel that his or her sexual and emotional needs are being met. If you have lost your desire for sex because sex was not enjoyable for you, you need to make an agreement with your partner to do what is necessary to make sex more pleasurable. Many of the exercises in this book will help you learn not only what it is that will bring you sexual pleasure but also how to make the necessary changes in your sexual relationship. If you want help with specific sexual complaints, such as an inability to reach orgasm or erection problems, turn to the Resources section at the end of this book.

Trauma

You may have answered true to some or all of the following questions: 20, 21, and 23.

Many women report having had uncomfortable, coercive, or unpleasant sexual encounters, especially as young women. The fact that there continues to be a high rate of sexual violence perpetrated against women and children is well documented. Current studies estimate that as many as one in five women has been sexually abused in childhood. About as many, 22 percent, report having been forced into some sexual activity by a man after the age of thirteen.[5] A history of sexual abuse and assault is frequently related to sexual desire problems in adulthood. It is only natural that there would be some fallout from these experiences. Marissa's story illustrates the long-term impact of a rape that she had thought was "past history."

By the time Marissa came for therapy, she had so many sexual rules for her husband to follow that she was not experiencing much sexual pleasure and had no sexual desire. The situation was extremely frustrating for both Marissa and for her husband, Frank. Neither could imagine anything in their relationship that would be responsible for Marissa's feelings. Marissa tentatively offered at the end of her first therapy session that she had been raped twenty years earlier, although she said she was sure this could not be related to her life now. With much embarrassment, Marissa told her story. When she was a freshman in college, she had gone out dancing with friends. After a few drinks, Marissa began talking and flirting with some of the guys at the bar, something she was normally too shy to do. Marissa was flattered when an attractive upperclassman began paying attention to her, buying her drinks, and holding her close to dance. She ignored her friends' warnings that he had a bad reputation; Marissa was attracted to him, she liked him, and she believed he liked her. Again ignoring her friends' cautionary advice, Marissa went back to his frat house. She anticipated fooling around but not having sex. After a couple of drinks in his room, Marissa awoke to find him on top of her having intercourse. When he was done, he returned her clothes and told her to leave. Upon leaving his room, she was greeted with catcalls and jeers from his roommates. For the rest of the year, Marissa was subjected to taunts from members of the frat house. She never told her friends what happened and transferred to another school the following year.

Even after twenty years and a happy marriage, Marissa blamed herself for the rape. Most specifically she blamed her sexual desire for getting her into a dangerous and humiliating situation. Twenty long years later, she had a profound mistrust of her sexual feelings and stayed disconnected from them at all costs.

Even if the situation is not a sexual assault as defined by law, many women have had sexual experiences that were humiliating to them, that they regretted, that were not in their best interest. Adolescent girls and young women typically view sex as a way to intimately connect and as a way to express intimate connection. Sexual contacts that result in unwanted pregnancy, a sexually transmitted disease, a rejection, or a betrayal can have a lasting impact on sexual desire. That teaches women to doubt and mistrust their sexual feelings. Without some insight most women will ultimately remain disconnected from their sexual desires. The negative sexual experiences of a close friend or a sister can have the same result. Women who work at rape crisis centers and shelters for abused women know that trauma can be vicariously experienced.

If you have been sexually abused or sexually assaulted, talking about it helps. Keeping it a secret allows the sense of shame to fester. If you are experiencing flashbacks (intrusive images or memories of the abuse), if you feel an aversion to sex or have panic attacks, consult a therapist before doing the work in this book. If you feel that the trauma is in the past but that sex has still been damaged, this book will be helpful to you as you reclaim your sexual desire. Specifically, the exercises that help you to focus on your conditions for sex and slowly getting in touch with your sexual desires can make sex a mutually pleasurable and desirable experience.

Abuse

(Read this if you even considered answering true to question 22.)

Sometimes lack of sexual desire is a sign that you are in a bad relationship and that physical intimacy should be avoided. It is not appropriate to feel sexually attracted to and interested in someone who treats you badly, belittles you, or abuses you. Often in abusive relationships, women's desires are not welcomed or considered. Iris's story highlights many of the issues that women struggle with when they are in a destructive relationship.

Iris was raised by strict parents who immigrated to the United States from Eastern Europe determined to become successful. They placed all of their hopes on their daughter, who, much to their disappointment, was not strong academically in the subjects they valued (mathematics, science). Iris's creativity and artistic ability were actively discouraged. Her parents were controlling and critical of her. As an adult Iris was attracted to controlling men. She mistook domination for caring. Ron, her current boyfriend, was not only controlling and critical but had a bad temper and was often verbally abusive. Ron had been physically abusive to his ex-wife and his children and often humiliated Iris in front of other people. He had even engaged in oral sex with his neighbor in front of Iris on a few occasions. He laughed at her and convinced her that she was being a prude when she voiced her objection. Iris attributed her lack of sexual desire to her menopausal age. This was one of a number of distorted beliefs Iris maintained in order to preserve the relationship. Iris felt trapped. Her friends and extended family were telling her that this was a bad relationship, and yet she loved Ron and did not want to be alone in the world.

For Iris and others like her, the problem is clearly not their lack of sexual interest but the poor quality of the relationship they are in. While it is beyond the scope of this book to help women end abusive relationships (either by ending the relationship altogether or by ending the abuse), women must attend to the message implicit in their lack of sexual desire. If you believe that your lack of desire is due to a bad relationship, ask yourself the following questions[6] and *pay attention to your answers.*

- Are you in a constant state of uncertainty and anxiety about what your partner wants or expects from you? Do you often feel as though you are walking on eggshells?

- Do you frequently worry about what mood your partner is in?

- Are you afraid of your partner's temper? Do you go along with what he wishes just to keep the peace?

- Is your partner excessively critical about even the little things? Does he humiliate or demean you?

- Does your partner make most or all of the decisions in the relationship (finances, friends, how to spend free time)?

- Do you feel that all the problems in the relationship are your fault, that your partner would be more loving if only you could get things right?

- Have you given up things of value or importance because your partner didn't like them or approve of them or forbade them (including friendships, time with your family, education, hobbies, leisure activities)?

- Do you ever feel physically threatened or intimidated by your partner?

- Has your partner ever pushed, kicked, slapped, or punched you? Has he ever thrown objects at you or used or threatened to use a weapon on you?

- Do you stay in the relationship because you do not want to be alone or are worried that no one else will want you or that your partner will hurt you if you leave?

If you answered yes to any of these questions, then your lack of desire may be a healthy response to an unhealthy relationship. You need to resolve the relationship issues first. Talk to family and friends about their perceptions of the relationship. Tell them what is going on so you can have an outside reality check. If the relationship is solid, it will stand up to scrutiny. Abuse festers in secret. Consider going into therapy with or without your partner. The Resources section at the end of this book will help you get started.

Depression

Depression is often cited as a factor in low sexual desire. Indeed, loss of libido is one of the symptoms of a clinical depression. Any and all of the imbalances mentioned in this chapter can lead to depression and, of course, loss of sexual passion. If you only treat the symptoms of depression and do not address the underlying cause, there will be no improvement in sexual desire. Trying to "treat the depression" without "treating the person" and her unique situation does not have good results. Sarah's story illustrates this point.

Sarah was a woman in her late twenties who was married for the second time and had no children. Sarah's husband was older than she was and was a police officer who, despite her objections, often worked long overtime hours. Sarah was concerned about the fact that she had little sexual desire for her husband. She worried that he might die in the line of duty and that she would not have been a good wife to him. So she asked her gynecologist about her low desire. The doctor heard "no sexual desire, depressed" and sent Sarah to a psychiatrist for medication. The psychiatrist prescribed Prozac, despite the fact that diminished sexual arousal is a frequent side effect. Sarah took Prozac for over a year. During that time she and her husband had more frequent sexual activity, but Sarah still felt no desire for sex. Her psychiatrist recommended adding Wellbutrin (an antidepressant with mild stimulating effects) to see if this would help increase her desire. It was at this point that Sarah stopped taking the Prozac and came to therapy. As she explained to me later, "If I have to use drugs to be interested in my husband, something is wrong."

Sarah was not happy with her life. She did not like the fact that her husband worked long hours and then volunteered for overtime. She did not like socializing only with other police officers and their wives. Her husband worried about her going out alone because of crime, and Sarah felt she had to go out either with her husband or not at all. When Sarah got in touch with the reason for her unhappiness and for her loss of desire, she began to make changes in her life. She began socializing with friends and took yoga classes twice a week in the evening. She asked her husband not to accept overtime unless he had to, and he acquiesced when he knew that Sarah would go out without him otherwise.

When Sarah felt that her life was more in her control and more reflective of her sensibilities, she did not feel depressed and she felt attracted to and interested in her husband again. As Sarah stated, "The Prozac just helped me accept a bad situation. I'm not sure that was a good thing."

Sarah's sadness and loss of desire were appropriate to her life situation. When she listened to her feelings, she was able to effectively address the problems that contributed to her unhappiness. Antidepressants can be helpful and appropriate in the treatment of depression. But not all feelings of sadness constitute a clinical depression, nor are all depressions effectively treated with medication. If you are depressed because something in your life is depressing you, address that problem (and this can involve going into therapy). If you cannot figure out why you are feeling depressed, consult a psychologist. Do not simply take antidepressant medication and expect improvement without making changes in your life. Medication should help you address your problems, not distract you from them.

Infidelity

An affair is almost always difficult to recover from. This is true regardless of whether it was you or your partner who had the affair. Among the common fallout from the discovery of an affair is a loss of sexual desire for the betraying partner. This may not happen immediately. The initial reaction of shock is often followed by a panic to hold on to the relationship and to regain the love feared lost. It makes intuitive sense that an affair should have a devastating effect on sexual desire. After all, the betrayal is of a sexual nature. Infidelity causes a breach of trust and so damages intimacy. It strikes at the heart of our feelings of self-worth and so damages our sexual self-esteem ("He prefers another lover to me—I'm not good enough for him.").

For many women an affair is traumatic, in the true sense of the word. It creates an emotional and psychological wound. Feelings of anger that we may not be comfortable sharing for fear of creating more distance in the relationship or pushing our partner into the arms of the other woman can lead to buried resentments.

The balance of power is often tipped toward the one threatening to leave, the one who appears to have other and better options. In other words, an affair can create disequilibrium in at least five out of the eight factors we have discussed (intimacy, sexual self-esteem, trauma, anger, and power). If you have discovered your partner being unfaithful to you more than once, you must consider that he likes keeping you off balance. It is up to you to decide whether you want to live this way. Hoping that he will change and that this affair will be the last is fruitless, unless your partner is expressing genuine remorse and is getting psychological help.

If this discovery of the affair is the only infidelity, you and your partner need to look at why such a breach of trust occurred. Remember, you are not to blame for your husband's or boyfriend's betrayal. Even if you both agree that the relationship has problems, there are other ways for someone to express his discontent. You share responsibility for the state of the relationship prior to the affair. You share responsibility for improving the relationship after the affair. Your partner needs to look at why he expressed his discontent in a way that injured you (and most likely the other woman as well). The story below illustrates just how destructive infidelity can be.

> Miriam discovered Steve's affair when she was looking for stamps in her husband's desk. Upon opening the drawer, she found a card from another woman thanking Steve for the best weekend of her life, a weekend during which Miriam was away visiting her sister. When confronted, Steve admitted that he had been corresponding with another woman over the Internet for more than a year and that they had met several times and had sex. Distraught, Miriam raged and interrogated Steve: when, where, how, and how often had they had sex? She tortured herself with all the details in an attempt to understand the betrayal. Steve left the house that night and stayed in a motel. He told Miriam he was going for good.
>
> Miriam alternated between anger and despair. She thought over the past year with Steve and wondered where she had failed him. She asked for, and got, a list of all her shortcomings. She begged Steve to return home and give her another chance, which he reluctantly agreed to do. For the next several weeks, Miriam cooked Steve's favorite foods, bought herself new clothes and sexy lingerie, and initiated sex with Steve every night. Miriam was determined to win Steve back and wondered what sort of vile woman would try to steal another woman's husband. One day while using the computer, Miriam discovered that her husband was still communicating with the other woman via e-mail and professing his love to her. Again Miriam confronted Steve, but this time she told him to get out.
>
> Steve and Miriam came to see me for help in resolving the

issue of whether to separate. They had a baby daughter, and their mutual love for her held them together. Through therapy Miriam and Steve decided they wanted to give their marriage another try. Steve broke off contact with his girlfriend and provided proof to his wife that he had done so. Steve also terminated the Internet connection to his computer. But with their new resolve came new problems. Miriam became increasingly angry with her husband, not only for the affair but also for how he had continued it even when she was trying hard to prove her worth to him. Whenever they had sex, Miriam had unwanted thoughts and images of her husband with the other woman. Soon she lost all sexual desire for him. Miriam's heightened sexual activity with Steve was driven by a panicked wish to prove to him that she was the better choice of sex partner for him. Once this panic subsided, Miriam was left with a kind of posttraumatic reaction that included intrusive and anxiety-provoking thoughts of his infidelity. Indeed, even outside the bedroom, Miriam became upset at any reference to things that reminded her of her husband's affair.

An affair takes time to recover from, and trust often takes longer to rebuild than to build in the first place. If your partner has had an affair, remember your rights.

- You have the right to demand that all contact with the other woman be terminated.

- You have a right to see proof that there has been no contact. You can look at credit card receipts, phone bills, and so on.

- You are entitled to have little trust in your partner and to take the time you need to heal.

- You have a right to love your partner again and trust him again. You do not have to leave him or dwell on the affair interminably.

- You can choose to forgive (or not).

- You must address the issues in your relationship that preceded and followed the affair.

If you are the one who has had an affair, is having an affair, or is considering having an affair, there are also things for you to think about. One is the strong possibility that you are mistaking the obsessive fantasy love that an affair promises for the real thing. There is no way your husband or steady boyfriend can compete with the thrill and excitement of an affair. The very forbidden and risky nature of an affair makes it thrilling. You may also be looking for a way out of your present relationship. Of course, it is possible that your new love is a better life choice for you. While most affairs do not lead to marriage, some do. You may need some time apart from both your lover and your husband to think through your decision. Counseling or therapy is a good option.

If you have chosen to give up the affair or if the affair ended for other reasons, you may be reading this book in the hopes of restoring passion in your marriage or current relationship. You may need some time to mourn the love lost. But if you are resolved to improve your current relationship, then it must be your focus. If you were once sexually attracted to your partner, there is a good chance that your sexual relationship can be rekindled. Whether you opt to tell your partner about the affair is a matter for you to decide. While it is important to be honest, you need to balance the honesty with a regard for your partner's feelings. The essential thing, if you are serious about working on your current relationship, is to terminate all contact with your lover (or prospective lover).

Affairs can arise from and create many of the imbalances responsible for a lack of passion in a relationship. They also pull on the desire for obsessive love that we have been led to believe is real, true love. In this day of Internet access, many people who would otherwise never take the opportunity to meet and develop another relationship now do so. The Internet in its anonymity appears harmless at first, but, paradoxically, for many people a chat room can become the place that holds out the promise of intimacy. If you find yourself "chatting" with a man and revealing more of your inner self to him than to your partner, go back and read the section on intimacy.

4

Taking Stock:
What Are You Saying
When You Are Saying No?

My unhappiness was the unhappiness
of a person who could not say no.

OSAMU DAZAI

As we read in the previous chapter, we lose sexual desire when an important part of our life is out of balance. As many of you will have discovered from answering the questions in Chapter 3, the imbalance is rarely restricted to one area. It may have started out that way, but, as we will learn in this chapter, it is difficult to limit the impact of any sexual problem to just one aspect of your life. Don't fool yourself into believing that your sexual disinterest is not that big a deal, that it is only a phase, or that you are making it up to yourself and your partner in other ways. Just as imbalances in your life can lead to decreased desire, decreased desire can upset the balance in your life. Alice and Richard's story is an example.

When Alice consulted me, her marriage of twenty-four years was coming to an end. Her husband, Richard, had told her that he could no longer live in a marriage without sex. He was approaching fifty and felt as though time was running out for him. Her husband's unhappiness was not news to Alice. Richard had complained about the sporadic and infrequent nature of their sexual relationship for years. He had tried many times to make changes. He had read books about sex, had planned romantic dinners, weekends away, brought flowers home, and in desperation went to therapy alone, because Alice wouldn't join him. Alice knew that her husband was unhappy about their lack of a sexual relationship, but she never believed that Richard would leave her. She had been a good friend and companion and had indulged many of his whims as an expression of her love. She was desperate to do something. The problem was that Richard felt it was too late. He had heard the promises before. Alice begged her physician to prescribe medication for her, but with her family history of breast cancer, she wasn't a good candidate for hormonal treatments. The problem was so much larger than any pill could handle. They went to therapy together, where Alice divulged that her beloved father had been arrested for exhibitionism when she was a young girl and that throughout her teen years her parents had fought about her father's deviant sexual behavior. Knowing why Alice did not view sex in a positive light, or see it as part of a loving marriage, was helpful to both Alice and Richard. However, a lot of damage had been done to the relationship by this point. Richard was not optimistic. He was hurt deeply by Alice's disinterest in him. After years of disappointment, Richard no longer felt interested in having sex with Alice. The prospect of rejection was just too great.

How Did We Get Here?

It is always a mistake to be indifferent to your partner's needs, no matter how trivial or unrealistic they may seem. Many women are dismissive of men's sexual interest. Perhaps women are simply worn out from years of listening to boys and then men talking about their sexual needs. Or perhaps women want to justify their own position that sex is just not that important. Women don't want to believe that they are letting their partners or themselves down in any truly significant way. Some women, especially those with low sexual self-esteem, believe that men's sexual desire exists in a universe of its own: "It's not me he wants, he just wants sex." Anna, whom we met in previous chapters, held on to the belief that her husband's sexual desire had little or nothing to do with her. In one of our first meetings, Anna explained that her husband had married her only for sex. Now, no one really has to get married to have sex, unless he or she is following strict religious proscriptions. And Anna was not even having sex with her husband! Either he was a complete fool or Anna was mistaken. Indeed, it was Anna's assumption that she needed to give men a reason (sex) to be with her. Her husband was stuck between a rock and a hard place. Paradoxically, the only way for him to show her he loved her was to leave her alone. What started off as an issue with low self-esteem developed into an unhealthy pattern of sexual disinterest.

The Downward Spiral

There is a great deal of support for the belief that men are interested in sex and not relationships. Didn't many of us get this warning from our parents when we began to date? Implicitly or explicitly, girls are given the message that boys and men are out for "one thing only." This belief makes it much easier to trivialize men's sexual interests throughout life. More "important" things like work, family obligations, and household chores can easily take precedence in our stress-filled lives.

When your husband or boyfriend approaches you for sex and you are tired, preoccupied, busy, and disinterested, you will wonder what is turning him on. As you assess the situation, you will find it highly unlikely that you are so sexy when you are cutting up vegetables for dinner, hunched over the computer doing bills, or fast asleep in bed that the sight of you has aroused great passion in him. You will conclude, "He is not interested in me. If he were, he would help prepare the dinner, leave me alone to do the bills, or let me sleep. He is being selfish. He just wants sex, and it has nothing to do with me." Your response to his sexual advance is likely to be no. But from your partner's perspective, the situation looks very different. He wants to have sex. You are his sexual partner. He would love it if you would stop whatever you are doing to have passionate sex with him. It would make him feel desired. It would result in his feeling closer to you, loved by you, valued by you. When you say no to him (again), he will feel hurt and rejected. Either he will avoid you and all intimate contact with you or he will pursue you even more doggedly. Whichever his response, the relationship is on a downward spiral. It is a pattern of "rejection ——➤ avoidance" or one of "rejection ——➤ pursuit ——➤ stronger rejection ——➤ stronger pursuit."

Regardless of which pattern occurs, you are likely to feel even more strongly that "all he wants is sex." In the first scenario, this belief is bolstered by the fact that your partner does not engage with you intimately in other areas of your life. In the second scenario, your partner's dogged pursuit of you feels obsessive, and you can easily believe that all he wants is sex.

Stopping the downward spiral long enough to gain some balance is part of the solution. In this chapter you will get the tools to evaluate the status of your present relationship, to assess the impact of your lack of interest, and to evaluate the strengths that you can build on.

The MUSIC Method

To help you examine the impact of your sexual disinterest on yourself, your partner, and your relationship, think of music. In any performance, there may be much that is right, but just one or two off-key notes or off-tempo beats can render a good piece of music bad. MUSIC is the acronym that I use to help couples explore their relationship. The letters stand for *Me, U (You), Sex, Intimacy,* and *Communication.* These five elements are the keys to a harmonious relationship. Each element is affected when there are problems in a relationship—for our purposes sexual problems. Each can also either contribute to or detract from your level of sexual desire. Asking women to check in and evaluate the impact of their low desire on the building blocks of their relationship often has a profound impact. Many women mistakenly believe that their low sexual desire can be compartmentalized off from the rest of their lives. Like Alice, they're shocked when confronted with just how damaging one's low sexual desire can be and how it can erode self-confidence (yours and his), create and maintain emotional distance, and interfere with healthy communication.

It is important to take some time at the beginning of your journey toward reclaiming your sexual desire to examine the impact of your low desire on the essential foundation of your relationship and your sense of self. This eye-opening experience can be extraordinarily motivating. Through it you'll recognize and and understand that you are working to reclaim your sexual passion for yourself and not simply to placate or silence your unhappy partner.

Many women do not believe that their lack of sexual interest affects them, except to the extent that their partner's unhappiness leads to arguments and tension in the relationship. Underneath it all, many of these women believe that everything would be fine if their husbands could just get over their adolescent fixation with sex. A great deal of marital tension results from the struggle over who is right, whose idea will prevail. She is struggling to prove to him that sex is not the most important part of the marital relationship. He is striving to prove that sex is vitally important. Both positions are valid and not mutually exclusive, but each battle pushes the couple further apart, until the battle has taken on a life of its own and no one is really sure what it is all about.

M—Me

The myth that "I am not affected by my lack of sexual interest" bears additional examination. Apart from whatever strife it engenders in a relationship, we can begin this exploration by asking ourselves, "What does my lack of sexual interest say about me?" The answers are often surprising. Some typical responses I have heard from my patients fall into one (or more) of the following four categories:

1. *There is something wrong with me (hormonally or psychologically).*

   - "My hormones are just out of whack."

   - "Since this happens in every significant relationship, I guess I have a problem being intimate."

   - "It makes me wonder if I am in love with my husband, but that makes me feel bad about myself. My husband is actually a pretty good guy. I wonder what is wrong with me that I wouldn't love him anymore."

   - "Sex is really no fun for me. But that must make me some sort of freak. Everyone else seems to think it is the greatest thing."

   - "When I hear a joke about sex, I feel like I have no right to laugh. I feel like a fraud."

   - "It makes me feel like a really terrible person. I know that my boyfriend would be ecstatic if I had the feeling back, but I just can't. I guess I feel kind of hopeless about the whole thing."

2. *I am old (chronologically, hormonally, psychologically).*

   - "I'm a mother now, and sex just can't be a priority. My kids are my life."

   - "I used to want to have sex a lot, but that was when I was younger. I guess I really feel that I'm too old for that kind of feeling."

   - "It's just menopause. All my friends are going through the same thing."

3. *I am sexually unattractive (sex is for the thin, beautiful, childless).*

   - "I'm too fat. I don't want my husband or anyone to see me naked."

   - "I guess I'm just not very sexy."

4. *I am not in control of my life (my schedule, my partner).*

- "I'm just too busy and too tired. There's simply no time for it."
- "I think my lack of sexual desire is pretty appropriate to my situation. I just can't be interested in a man who treats me the way my husband does. Of course, I feel responsible for this as well. After all, I chose to marry him. I made a bad decision, and now I'm stuck with it."
- "My husband thinks he can just roll over and grab me. And this is after a day of him grousing about everything or, worse, ignoring me. I know he's really busy and his job is very stressful, but I can't seem to make him understand that his behavior affects me and my sex drive!"

Women's responses to this question highlight the reality that one's level of sexual desire has important implications on how one views oneself. Now ask yourself, "How do I *want* to feel about me?" For many women the answer can be summarized by the following statements:

- I'm happy. I'm in control of my life, and I'm where I want to be, or I'm on the way.
- I'm healthy and well adjusted (physically and mentally). I'm normal.
- I'm attractive.
- I'm young. If not in years, then I'm young at heart. I have retained my youthful energy and enjoyment of life.

Certainly I am not arguing that women can change the way they feel about themselves solely by increasing their level of sexual interest. What I do want to emphasize is that your level of sexual interest has an impact on your sense of self and that addressing your sexuality can be an important part of improving your overall self-image. Instead of staying stuck believing that "when I feel better about myself, I can improve my sex life," entertain the idea that you can approach it from the opposite perspective: "When I improve my sex life, I will feel better about myself."

U—*You*

Let's face it. Your lack of sexual interest not only says something about how you think and feel about yourself, it also speaks to how you think and feel about your partner. Most women do not intend their sexual disinterest to be hurtful to their partners. In cases of unresolved anger, or where the balance of power is clearly tipped in his favor, withholding sexual desire can be a powerful weapon, the ace up your sleeve. You may be tempted to use it as such.

There are two very important reasons that this is not a good strategy for addressing the problems in your relationship. First, withholding sexual desire rarely addresses the real problem, but it can compound an already bad situation. The original problem festers, and the relationship suffers from two blows instead of one. The second reason has to do with collateral damage to your own and your partner's sense of self-esteem and competence. As we've seen, low sexual desire takes its toll on women. It also takes its toll on men.

Whether it is intended or not, the message men get when their partners have little sexual desire is, "There's something wrong with you." So while women often blame themselves for their lack of desire, men hear a different message. What men hear can fall into one of the following four categories:

1. *You are not lovable.*
   - "Honestly, I feel like a jerk. Especially around other guys."
   - "I'm not sure I'm answering the question exactly. But it makes me feel hopeless, like we'll never get back to the way it used to be—you know, when we were in love."
   - "She doesn't love me anymore."
2. *You are not a priority in my life.*
   - "I feel that all I am is a workhorse. I go to work. I help with the kids. I work around the house. I take care of the cars. Frankly, I don't feel appreciated."
   - "I don't buy that there is no time. She has time for everything but sex."

3. *You are not sexually desirable./You are not a good lover.*
   - "I feel like my father."
   - "I guess I'm no Don Juan."

4. *You are too needy.*
   - "I feel like a dog begging for table scraps. I mean, c'mon, she never wants to have sex with me, and when we do have sex, I feel like she's doing me a big favor."
   - "Well, I get the feeling she thinks I'm a pervert or something."

Looking over this list, most of us recognize that these are not the messages we intend to give our partners, though this is clearly what they hear.

When your sexual disinterest gives your partner the message that there is something wrong with him, he may act defensively and tell you that there is something wrong with you. When I originally met Anna, she was worn out from the constant arguments that ultimately ended with Brian's exhorting her to "fix her problems." In self-defense Anna viewed Brian in a negative light: "He has such a bad temper. He's forgetful and neglectful. It's no wonder I don't want to have sex with him!" Anna would recount the arguments to her friends, who would reinforce her belief that Brian's behavior was responsible for pushing her away sexually and otherwise. Anna and Brian were locked in a battle over who was right, and while they were busy defending their positions, they were doing nothing to make their marriage better.

If we want to preserve the relationship, we may try to demonstrate our affection and regard in other ways. Donna laid out her husband's clothes for him each day, being careful that everything would match. Jennifer continued to try to be the perfect wife and mother, preparing good meals and keeping the house clean. Alice (whom we met at the beginning of this chapter) indulged her husband's other desires. She devoted a large part of the household budget to making the payments on her husband's sailboat. However, each of these remedies did nothing to alleviate the tension caused by the sexual disinterest. Indeed, each of these women chose a remedy that actually contributed to the imbalance in their lives. Donna continued to put her husband's interests above her own, paying more attention to his clothing than to her own. Jennifer's perfectionism only added to her stress, and Alice acted on her belief that sex did not have to be an important part of the relationship. However, when all is said and done, Donna, Jennifer, and Alice (and others like them) will feel resentful when their loving gestures do little to improve their husbands' mood or the tenor of the relationship. And so the downward spiral continues.

Positive Messages   It is essential to give some consideration to how you would like to think about your partner and the message you would like to convey to him. Anna summarized her thoughts on the subject quite nicely:

> I love Brian. I would like to believe that I made the right decision when I married him. I would like to believe that although he is not perfect, he is a good partner for me. Most of all I want to believe that he loves me and that his sexual desire is an expression of his love for me.

If you are committed to staying in your current relationship, give some thought to your partner's positive aspects as well as to the message you would like to convey to him regarding your feelings for and about him.

When You Think Your Partner Has a Problem   The message that our partner is fundamentally a good and lovable man is one that conveys a healthier respect for our partners and ourselves. Conveying this message becomes difficult when we are really angry with our partner or when there is an underlying sexual problem. In the first instance, we can look at Lorna and Tom's situation. As you may recall, Lorna had a great deal of anger at Tom for changing his job without consulting her. His apology had effectively cut off further discussion.

Lorna continued to be furious with Tom and found every opportunity to berate him and point out his shortcomings. In therapy Lorna focused her anger on two things: first on the hurt she felt that he had disregarded her in an important decision (the job) and second on how his behavior cut her off from expressing her feelings. When Lorna and Tom finally had a few difficult but productive discussions about the manner in which Tom had changed jobs, Lorna stopped seeing him in such a negative light. She was still often angry with him for things he did, but she was not angry with him for who he was. This change allowed Lorna to see Tom in a more positive light and to have some positive and sexual feelings for him. He didn't have to be perfect to be lovable.

When your partner has a sexual dysfunction, the issue again becomes clouded. How do you convey to someone that there is nothing wrong with him when neither of you believes it? This was a problem that Mindy and Calvin encountered.

Mindy did not know how to talk openly to Calvin about his premature ejaculation. However, it was not a secret to Calvin that this problem cut short their lovemaking. Though Mindy did not complain, Calvin could sense her frustration. Every time Calvin wanted to have sex and Mindy put him off, he felt like a loser. Every time he ejaculated quickly and Mindy told him it was okay, he felt inept and inadequate. Both Mindy and Calvin knew that it was *not* okay. When Mindy and Calvin went to therapy, they learned that a pattern of rapid ejaculation is often learned in adolescence. When they understood that ejaculatory control can be developed in adulthood, they no longer viewed Calvin as sexually inept.

Your lack of sexual interest in your partner communicates a broader disinterest in him. Your partner will feel wounded and hurt by your refusal to have sex with him or by your lack of enthusiasm for sex with him. This message gets conveyed even if you take all the blame on yourself—"It's not you, it's me." There may be things about your partner that you want him to change. There may be things that your partner does or does not do that turn you off. By not addressing these issues, but instead letting your disinterest speak for you, you are sending a message that you may not mean to send. Although you may wish he were, your partner is not a mind reader. He cannot know, if you do not tell him, what you need and want to change in order to bring about a return of your desire. Not only do you need to be clear, you need to convey your message in a loving manner, without blame. Talking about sexual problems in the middle of sex or in the middle of an argument is never a good idea. In Chapter 7 you will find more guidance as to how to communicate effectively with your partner about difficult sexual issues.

S—Sex

Many women who complain of low sexual desire strongly believe that sex is too big an issue in their relationship, that it is too big a deal. Often they're right! However, many women mistakenly believe that the solution is to shrink sex down to its rightful place by minimizing it, trivializing it, or ignoring it. They are then surprised when the problem seems to grow bigger and more out of control. There is a wonderful children's book titled *There's No Such Thing as a Dragon*,[1] which illustrates this very point. It's a story about a boy who discovers a tiny dragon in his bedroom one morning. When all the adults refuse to believe in dragons and convince the boy to do the same, the tiny dragon grows bigger and bigger, until he occupies the entire house. Finally everyone acknowledges the presence of the dragon, and immediately the unwieldy beast shrinks back down to size. If discussions about sex or arguments about sex or even the avoidance of sex occupies a great deal of your emotional energy, then try giving sex its due. Acknowledge to your partner and yourself that sex is an important issue in your relationship.

Your sexual disinterest conveys the following messages:

- Sex is not an important part of a relationship.
- Sex is not important to me.

- Good relationships are strong enough to withstand interruptions—even long ones—in sexual activity.

- Sexual passion naturally dies out in a long-term relationship.

- Sex is natural; you cannot force it or work on it. Either sexual feelings are there or they are not.

You may reject some or all of these messages when they are stated so bluntly. But make no mistake: your sexual disinterest is broadcasting these messages loud and clear. In turn these messages reinforce and justify your low desire. Consider the opposing views for a moment:

- Sex is an important part of a relationship.

- Being sexual is important to me.

- Even good relationships are damaged when sexual activity is interrupted.

- Sexual passion can thrive in a long-term relationship.

- Sexual expression is learned. You definitely have to work on it in order to keep the feelings alive.

If these were the beliefs you held, sexual avoidance fed by sexual disinterest would be much less acceptable to you. But of course many women with low sexual desire continue to have sex for their partner's benefit. Donna continued to have sex with her husband because she felt that it was her place to fulfill all his needs. What she did not understand was that he was not interested in what I call "obligatory sex" and what is sometimes more crudely referred to as "mercy sex" or a "pity f——k."

So here's the good news and the bad news: Even if you are having sex despite your disinterest, it conveys a message to your partner. If he cares about you and the quality of the relationship, he will not be satisfied with obligatory sex. If he doesn't care about you and doesn't want sex to be a connecting experience . . . well then, by all means lie back and think of England. Or better yet think of a way out of this bind. Now, this is not to say that you should never be motivated to have sex by a desire to make your partner happy. But obligatory sex is not that kind of sex. It doesn't make your partner happy. It just feeds the myth that he is a needy person who must be placated. It also perpetuates the imbalance between your needs and his. More about this kind of sex—and how to break out of it—in the next chapter.

I—Intimacy

Avoiding sex means avoiding your partner, and this necessarily makes intimacy impossible. Jennifer, who felt tremendous stress after the birth of her daughter, did not want to argue with her husband about sex. She wanted him to understand, without her having to explain it, that she did not have the energy for sex. Because Jennifer wanted to avoid sex and avoid arguments or discussions about it, she began to avoid her husband.

> My husband likes to watch the evening news. I am too tired, so I go up to bed before he does. Most nights I am asleep before Bill makes it up the stairs, but sometimes I am still awake, thinking about what I need to do the next day. But the thing is, I pretend to be asleep. I haven't done that since I was a kid. I pretend to be asleep, and I pray that Bill won't reach over for me. Most of the time I'm hugging my side of our queen-size bed, and we don't even touch. I relax when I can tell he is asleep. In the mornings I'm out of bed like a shot. During the day I tense up when Bill approaches me. I don't want to hug for too long, or he might get the wrong idea. I don't even like to talk affectionately, because I don't want to raise the issue of sex. Of course, every now and then I get nervous and tell Bill I love him, and I want to hear that he loves me, too. When he says it, I heave a huge sigh of relief. We're okay. Then it starts all over again.

Jennifer's story is certainly not unique. Intimate connections are very difficult to maintain when a relationship gets out of balance. The real tragedy is that the relationship is further imbalanced as couples struggle to deal with one partner's lack of sexual interest. Sex becomes a burden, a topic of contention. Anna's view that her husband married her just for sex got reinforced as the frequency of their lovemaking declined. Whenever Brian approached Anna, he was open to the possibility of having sex. He longed for and watched for any sign of thaw in her demeanor toward him. Thus begins a familiar refrain. Women complain that their husbands never touch them except when they want sex. Men complain that they never get sex. In truth, when sex is an integrated part of a relationship, intimate touching is a way to remind each other of the connection.

The bottom line is that sex is a vital part of an intimate relationship. Its importance is determined by how well it fits into the larger whole of your relationship, rather than how often you have it. When sex is problematic, it drains off a huge proportion of the energy within a relationship. When sex is a natural part of the relationship, its importance is simply understood and difficult to parcel out. As a good friend of mine once remarked when she was talking about her partner, "It's fun to be lovers." In an increasingly complicated and stressful world, we do need a little fun.

C—Communication

As you may have gathered by now, when you avoid sex, you are communicating more than a sexual disinterest to your partner. You are telling him that neither he nor sex is a priority for you. Being aware of the messages you are sending can help you to understand your partner's reactions and can help you choose more consciously the message you would like to convey.

Many people think of talking as the only means of communication. Certainly it can be one of the clearest forms. But talking about sex— putting your feelings into words and being concerned about your partner's reaction—makes verbal communication in this realm very difficult for most women. We have little practice honestly communicating about sex. Sex education is a misnomer. In most sex-ed classes, there is very little education about sex going on. We're taught the consequences of sex, the biology of reproduction, and in more liberal areas the mechanics of contraception. The mechanics of the sex act itself are conveniently left out. The message that we have received is that sex should come naturally to us, that we should just be good at it. So when sex becomes a problem, we find ourselves without the tools to talk about it.

One very major source of miscommunication arises from touch. Women who are avoiding sex are vigilant to any sexual overtures. Perhaps hypervigilant. If you are avoiding sex, you will respond to all intimate touch as though it were a sexual invitation. This means that you will in some way reject physical intimacy, which will inevitably lead to less and less physical contact and more emotional space or distance between you and your partner.

If all touch doesn't necessarily lead to sex (and it doesn't), then how do we know what is a prelude to sex? And what kind of sex is it a prelude to? The success of evasive maneuvers around the initiation of sex makes the interested party more blunt and more direct. As a result a woman will often complain that the manner in which her lover proposes sex turns her off: "There's no romance, no seduction." Or he doesn't initiate at all. This leaves the disinterested woman in a very awkward situation. She believes she knows when her husband or boyfriend wants sex. She may believe he wants it all the time or on particular occasions (after an evening out, when the kids have gone to sleep over at friends'). In any event it leaves her either to propose something she is not interested in or spend the time as though she were walking on eggshells, saying without saying, "I know I am disappointing you, but I really don't feel like having sex."

Low sexual desire creates or contributes to communication problems in the relationship. Sex becomes a contentious issue; emotional intimacy and intimate touch are avoided. The negative messages that are conveyed do not get clarified. Sex becomes more of an obligation, not something we may be open to or even desirous of. It becomes less mutual and less negotiable. It's all his way or nothing. Communication problems can contaminate other areas of our relationship, and, like Jennifer, we may stop talking affectionately to our partner. We may avoid discussions of other difficult subjects.

Listening to the MUSIC

When we tune in to the MUSIC of our relationship, we can more fully understand how our sexual disinterest distorts our interactions and creates bad feelings (for both partners) and distance between would-be lovers. With this realization we can be more fully motivated and committed to making the changes necessary to reclaim our sexual passion. While it is certainly an option to fix all the problems in one's relationship with the expectation that passionate feelings will follow, this approach rarely works well. Sexual problems and relationship problems coexist and feed off each other. Addressing your sexual disinterest necessarily means addressing issues in your relationship—and vice versa. When you listen to the MUSIC of your relationship, you will become aware of the changes you need to make.

5

Reclaiming Your Sexual Self

A woman doesn't fall in love with a man's need.
She falls in love with his need for her.

ROSEMARY SULLIVAN

Implicit in the definition of desire is the fact that one must want something for oneself. Women who lack desire do not think of sex as something for them. They think of it as something they do for someone else. An important step in reclaiming desire is believing that sex is something worth wanting, that sex is something that is good for you. But as girls we certainly did not get this message. Girls are rarely told the joys and benefits of good sex. Sex-education classes are filled with the dangers but not the pleasures of sex. For example, most drawings of the female genitalia in sex-education texts omit the clitoris. If it is included and if it is labeled, its function (solely for pleasure) is not explained. It would appear that telling girls that sex can be pleasurable for them is strictly taboo. However, as young women we are bombarded with messages that we should be good at sex. There is not a month that goes by that a women's magazine does not run some article called "How to Drive Your Man Wild in Bed." Advice columns and books for women interested in getting into a committed relation-

82

ship instruct the reader as to the strategic importance of when to have what level of sexual activity. The object is to snag the man, not to see if your intimacy can translate into satisfying sex. Many of my clients have complained that their early upbringing led them to think that sex was not good *for* them only to discover that as young women it was something they were supposed to be good *at*. We were not encouraged as girls to understand and explore the physical sensations that our sexual thoughts might have inspired. We were not given permission to revel in the physical sensations that may have come with sexual activity by ourselves or with someone else. For many women the message that we should put our own needs, wants, aspirations, and ambitions aside when we love someone makes it difficult to stay in touch with our sexual feelings, especially when those physical feelings of sexual excitement are not as strong as they once were.

In her book *The Mismeasure of Women,* the social psychologist Carol Tavris describes her delight and confusion when as a child she saw the musical *Annie Get Your Gun.* The story, as some of you may know, involves Annie Oakley, a woman who rode horses and could shoot better than any man, including her rival, Frank Butler. At the end of the musical, Annie, realizing that she loves Frank, intentionally loses her next competition with him. He then realizes he loves her, and we are into happily-ever-after territory. The real story, as Dr. Tavris points out, is that Frank Butler fell in love with Annie Oakley after she beat him. Far from giving up her life as a sharpshooter (or intentionally throwing matches), Annie went on to star in Buffalo Bill's Wild West show, and Frank became her manager and her husband. But the real story—a man in love with a woman more talented than he—was not the stuff of fairy tales—or musicals, although the story of a woman's sacrificing her talents and her career for the love of a man apparently is. We don't have to look as far as Broadway or Hollywood to find more examples of a woman who sacrifices some important part of her self (intelligence, competence, career) in order to win the affections of a man. Who among us has not feigned ignorance or pretended to need help when it was not really necessary, in order to appeal to a boy or a man? We may feel that we are making small sacrifices for peace or the sake of our partner's ego, but when this sacrificial attitude is applied to sex, it is a sure recipe for losing desire.

Obligatory Sex

We have seen that avoiding sex has some serious negative consequences for our relationships. Many women, wanting to avoid arguments and conflict, will have sex with their partner even though they
have no real desire to do so. But there are also problems with applying
Nike's "just do it" approach to sex. When having sex has nothing to
do with your own needs or wants, you will become further disconnected from your own sexual desire. Donna's story illustrates this
point.

> Both Donna and Michael had become accustomed to her lack of
> interest, which meant that their lovemaking had become per-
> functory. He did not spend much time or energy trying to please
> Donna sexually, because most of the time she wasn't interested
> and they would both be frustrated by his efforts. Donna concen-
> trated on pleasing Michael, which she believed meant stimulat-
> ing him to orgasm. When Michael would insist that he wanted
> Donna to experience pleasure, too, Donna would use her vibra-
> tor. Not only did she equate pleasure with orgasm, but she also
> felt extremely uncomfortable with the amount of time it would
> take her to climax without this mechanical device. On occasion
> Donna did feel some sexual interest, but she didn't know how
> she could say, "Okay, this time I'm really interested, and I would
> like to get more aroused, too." To say this would be to acknowl-
> edge her disinterest at other times when she had assured Michael
> that everything was fine for her. Donna kept trying to have sex at
> times and in ways she thought Michael wanted it. She continued
> to be dismayed that her passion and her pleasure were not
> greater. Michael continued to be dissatisfied with what he felt
> was simply obligatory sex.

Donna's story may represent a rather extreme version of what happens in many bedrooms across the country on a nightly basis: women
having sex solely to please their partners. Donna is not unique in this
"me second" approach to relationships. Many women get trapped in
this same conundrum. They feel they must satisfy all their partner's

needs and put their own on hold. This feeling is only deepened by the awareness that their partner is unhappy sexually. When a woman doesn't feel sexual desire, she will want to make it up to her partner to please him or to alleviate her own sense of guilt. So she thinks that she will have sex for her partner's sake soon. The problem with this type of thinking is that it takes women further from their own feeling of desire and closer to that suffocating sense of obligation. The message that is being promoted is that "I have to have sex with my partner to make him happy, to keep the peace, to avoid an argument, to alleviate my guilty feelings, to make me feel like a good partner, so he doesn't look elsewhere. . . ."

Where does this take us? If most or all of the time that women are having sex they are doing it for any or all of the above stated reasons, the sex is not likely to be too great—for them. Lack of sexual enjoyment can become a vicious cycle: she doesn't expect much from sex, she and her partner don't put much energy into pleasing her sexually, and as a result she doesn't get much pleasure from sex. Women who are stressed by the many demands placed upon them with little or no time to spare often fall into this same trap. The desire to "accomplish sex" detracts from any passionate connection that can be made. Remember Jennifer, who decided whether or not to have sex based on the number of hours she would still have to sleep? She clearly found herself caught in a cycle of disappointing sex.

> Jennifer was tired most of the time. When her husband reached out for her at night, she usually had a sinking feeling. She wanted to sleep, but she wondered how many more times could she put Bill off before a huge fight ensued. More often than she liked to admit, Jennifer responded to Bill with a businesslike agenda: make him happy as quickly as possible and get back to sleep. Occasionally Jennifer felt herself becoming aroused. Sometimes she would go with it, and sometimes she would not. Again, her decisions were primarily based on her competing desire for sleep. Sex with her own arousal factored in would usually take more time. When she did respond sexually to Bill's caresses, Jennifer found herself feeling happy and emotionally close to her husband. She would resolve that she would engage in and enjoy

sex more often. But her resolve never lasted. To avoid more fights or bad feelings, Jennifer would fall back upon the perfunctory, obligatory sex, when in reality she didn't want to have sex at all.

What both of these couples and many more like them have in common is an imbalance in the focus of their sexual energies. For Donna and Jennifer, the primary reason for having sex was to satisfy the partner, or at least each came to act as though her partner's sexual satisfaction was paramount *and took precedence over her own needs and wishes.* From such a position, it is not a stretch to get to the point where sex becomes an obligation or a duty, and obligatory sex kills passion.

Many of the women described in this book were initially quite gratified and pleased with their partner's sexual interest and desire *for them.* Passion fuels passion. The troubles often started when the women began to have sex mostly to please their partner. They may have been angry, too tired, too stressed, or just not in the mood. But too many episodes of having sex when you don't really want to lead to the feeling that perhaps your partner's desire is not *for you* but simply to gratify a sexual need of *his.*

It is inevitable in any relationship, no matter how good it is, that there will come a time when one person will want to have sex and the other will not feel so inclined. *How these situations are handled is the important thing.* If you believe that your needs and wishes are secondary to your partner's (at least in terms of sex), then you may fall into the pattern of having recurrent episodes of obligatory and passion-defeating sex, as the diagram below illustrates.

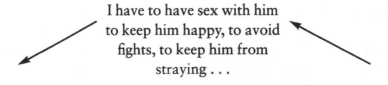

I have to have sex with him
to keep him happy, to avoid
fights, to keep him from
straying . . .

Since sex is not for me,
what we do sexually
will be for his pleasure.

Sex is not very
exciting for me./My pleasure
is not important.

As you can see from the diagram, many women begin to believe that their partner is not interested in their sexual pleasure.

Women who have been sexually abused as children already have this belief ingrained in them. Sexual acts between children and adults are never for the benefit of the child, no matter what pedophiles or child molesters may say. Such acts are for the sexual gratification of the adult. If you were abused as a child, it may be difficult to get to the point where you truly believe that your sexual pleasure is important to you and to your partner. Having sex solely for your partner's pleasure is perpetuating an old and maladaptive sexual pattern. Kendra's story is an example of this.

Kendra had been sexually abused by her father and her brothers. At the age of sixteen, she married to get out of the house, but her husband was physically abusive to her. When she finally left that marriage, she met and married Ted. Ted had never had a long-term relationship. He was shy and anxious and insecure around women. Kendra made him feel wonderful, and they had sex almost daily for the first two years of their relationship. However, once Ted was not interested in having sex so frequently, Kendra became highly anxious. Her anxiety would peak whenever she and Ted went more than a day without some sexual contact. Kendra's upbringing was an extreme example of the message that women exist to serve men's sexual needs. When Kendra and Ted finally made it to therapy, she revealed that she had no sexual desire and got little pleasure from sex. Sex was something she did almost compulsively in order to please her partner. She did not know what to make of the fact that Ted loved her and did not demand sex from her.

Many women have had early sexual experiences that did not constitute child abuse or rape but that nonetheless contributed to the belief that men primarily want sex from women. Too many girls have sex in an effort to establish a relationship, to keep a relationship, or to renew a relationship. Some even have sex to prolong a relationship that should by all rights be over. They are then left perplexed, thinking, "I had sex with him, and even then he didn't want me." Under these circumstances sex is not an intimate act but an instrumental act, a means to an end. Too many incidents of instrumental sex will take you further from being able to tune in to your own sexual desire. Instrumental sex in the beginning of a relationship can easily lead to obligatory sex later on.

Faking It

Many men tell their partner that her sexual pleasure is paramount. They may be sincere, or they may not. Their lover may believe them, or she may not. Often what you believe will be related more to your own history than to your partner's sincerity. (We will address the case of what happens when your partner truly is unconcerned about your pleasure later in this chapter.) What is certain is that women who fake interest, pleasure, or orgasm are buying in to the myth that men are really concerned only with satisfying their own ego.

Lonnie Barbach, who wrote *For Yourself*,[1] a guide to becoming orgasmic for women, noted that women commonly cope with the inability to reach orgasm by faking one. She listed three reasons that women faked orgasm:

1. So that their partners wouldn't think them inadequate
2. To protect a partner's ego
3. To get sex over with

But as Dr. Barbach points out, these women often find themselves stuck in the web of their own pretense. They may be so concerned with their "performance" that they tune out their own pleasure. Faking orgasms also gives your partner incorrect information about what turns you on. And finally, unless you are prepared to keep up the pretense indefinitely, we have the sticky question of how to stop faking.

How do you tell your partner that what he thought was turning you on all this time really is not? The best choice is never to pretend to have feelings, interests, and pleasures that you don't have. If that is no longer an option, your best bet is to acknowledge that you have been less than forthright about your interest, understanding that this information might hurt your partner's feelings. You should affirm your commitment to honesty in sexual matters in the future. You can stress that your intentions were honorable, although the means were not. Most important, you can take responsibility for your choice and your decision. Your partner did not make you fake an orgasm.

Telling your partner that things have changed and that what once turned you on no longer does is not a good option. It perpetuates the dishonesty in your sexual interactions, and it puts you in the position of defending yourself and your choices: "But why don't you like that anymore? Lets try it again! What's happened to you? You used to be so sexual!" Here are some tips on how to talk to your partner about faked or exaggerated pleasure:

- Tell your partner of your new intentions to be more present and genuine during sex.
- Be truthful about the fact that in the past you often gave the impression that you were more aroused than you were, and yes, that sometimes you know you gave the impression that you had an orgasm when you did not.
- Do not dwell on this. Do not answer all the questions about when and where you faked an orgasm and which ones were authentic and which ones were not. There is nothing to be gained by this. Keep asserting your commitment to be honest in all future sexual encounters. Know that you will have to rebuild the trust that has been damaged.
- Remember, your partner has suffered a blow to his ego. Reassure him that it is because you are interested in him sexually that you are able to be genuine with him.

It will take time, but this wound will heal, especially when you both experience just how connecting and intimate your sexual relationship will become. If you have difficulty reaching orgasm, or if you have never experienced an orgasm, you will find references to self-help books in the Resources section at the back of this book. For now, suffice it to say that you should not bring up the issue in anger or use it as a weapon to hurt your partner. Don't beat yourself up over this either.

You are in good company. The sex therapist Bernie Zilbergeld[2] once remarked that although 70 percent of women have faked an orgasm, 100 percent of people have faked feelings. What is important is your commitment to good sex and honesty in the future.

Your Sexual Satisfaction Counts

Many women are unaware of how important their pleasure is to their partner. For some men, their partner's pleasure reassures them about their masculinity, their desirability, and the security of the relationship. For many others, their sexual pleasure is enhanced because it is a shared pleasure. Donna didn't believe that her sexual desires were as important as Michael's. Jennifer thought Bill would be satisfied with obligatory sex, although she continued to feel that if he really cared about her, he would let her sleep. There is a qualitative difference between obligatory sex and mutually satisfying sex. And men who care know the difference.

But the real issue is whether we women care about it. If we care about our sexual pleasure and are unwilling to have perfunctory sex solely because someone else wants it, then our sex lives will necessarily change. Even when your partner is singularly focused on "getting off," you don't have to buy in to that. If you focus on your pleasure and on expanding the boundaries of what constitutes sex (kissing the neck or the ears, massaging the back, the feet, etc.), your partner may discover that getting it on is better than getting off. Going back to Brenda's story provides some helpful guidance.

Brenda had lost her sexual desire as a result of having mostly unsatisfying sex with her husband. Sex was mechanical and genitally focused. In bed Dennis would often just grunt and reach for Brenda by way of sexual initiation. He would grab her hand and place it over his erect penis. He would then direct her to touch or orally stimulate his penis for a few moments. Then they would have intercourse. Brenda tried talking to Dennis, tried explaining to him how she wanted to have sex. But there was not much change. There was a period of almost six months when Brenda even stopped having sex with Dennis, but this upset her as well. She wanted to have a sexual relationship with her husband. With some introspection Brenda realized that she had been passively waiting for Dennis to change. Finally she began acting as assertively in bed as she did out of it. She directed Dennis as he directed her. In time it wasn't such a struggle, although Brenda needed to continually direct Dennis and redirect him if he got too focused on orgasm. But their sex life vastly improved, and Dennis is appreciative. He knows that he can be too goal-oriented and that he needs a nudge every now and then to remind him that there is more to sex than "getting off." Brenda is much happier as well. She is now concentrating on trying to get Dennis to be more interactive outside of the bedroom.

Later chapters contain helpful tips on how to improve your sexual relationship. But first you have to get to the place where that appeals to you.

Attitude Is Everything

Attitudes shape and change our behavior if and only if our attitudes are directly relevant to the behavior we want to change. Having a positive attitude toward health and well-being does not necessarily translate into a desire to quit smoking. How many times have we been surprised by the athlete or the dancer who smokes? When someone's attitude about smoking changes, his or her smoking behavior changes.

So it is with sex. Our desire to have a good and harmonious relationship with our long-term partner does not in and of itself translate into an improvement in our sexual desire. As we have seen, the desire for a good relationship may result in someone's doing many things for the person she loves, including avoiding conflict. When your attitude about sex changes, only then will your sexual behavior and interest change. The following exercise will help you visualize how things could change for the better.

The Parallel-Universe Exercise

Imagine that you have found yourself in a parallel universe. Everything and everyone is the same—your husband, your kids (or lack thereof), your job, your living circumstances, everything—with one important exception. You have sexual desire in this parallel universe. To help you stay focused, it is best to write down your thoughts. Begin with the statement "I want to have sex with [name of your partner]." Now think about how this would change your reactions and interactions (both sexual and nonsexual) with your partner. Here are some questions to help you imagine how things would be different:

How does this change I how feel about him and about his desire?

How does this change the amount of contact I have with him?

How does this change how I feel about my relationship and myself?

How does this change how I feel about sex?

How does this change how I feel about the world around me?

Here's what Jennifer had to say when she did the exercise:

I want to have sex with Bill; therefore I would approach him more. Not just for sex, but I'd probably want to be around him. I guess I wouldn't work so much. If I wanted to have sex with Bill, he'd be a lot happier. I would be, too. I wouldn't think I'd have to make it up to him all the time by doing all the housework and cooking. That would be nice. Maybe if I stopped overcompensating, I would feel like I had the time to have sex! I would also be able to talk to Bill about some things that are bugging me. I never do, because I know he can always bring up the topic of sex, which I would do anything to avoid—in the old universe, that is. So I could talk to Bill more. That would make me feel a lot closer to him; in fact, we'd *be* a lot closer. That would be really nice. And I wouldn't be afraid to touch him anymore. If I weren't avoiding sex, I wouldn't avoid holding hands, being arm in arm, asking for my back to be scratched. This is a bit of a surprise, but I think I would feel younger and more attractive.

I would go out into the world of minivans and soccer moms with an inner grin: I have still got it. Gosh, I wish I wanted to have sex!

Wanting to want to have sex—it sounds somewhat odd, but it is a great starting point from which to work on your desire. The Parallel-Universe exercise also shows you just how much of an impact you can have on your life. The problem is not that your partner wants too much sex. Simply viewing your troubles in this way gives you little control over the outcome. So, armed with the knowledge that you can be responsible for drastically changing your sexual and romantic life, make a note of the reasons you found for wanting to want to have sex. Try to have at least three. Make sure that the reasons are for you and not just to make your partner happy. Remember, if you want to have an impact on your sexual desire, you must work specifically on your attitude toward sex with your current partner. Write down your reasons. Keep them near you—on your bedside table, next to your vitamins or your toothbrush, anywhere you will have the opportunity to look at them on a regular basis. And by all means *do* look at them on a regular basis.

Remember that wanting to have desire is different from actually having it. Your wish to have desire also needs to be oriented toward the future and not the past. The desire you get will not necessarily feel like the desire you had as an adolescent or the passion you felt in the beginning of your relationship. It may have much more of an emotional feel to it, rather than being a strong physical urge. Think of desire as the willingness or the readiness to connect intimately with your partner. The physical arousal and desire may be experienced only once you have begun making love. Anna's story provides a good example of how to use your new definition of desire:

Anna only engaged in obligatory sex, as she felt no desire for sex at all. Her inevitable response to Brian's sexual invitations was invariably no. She had, however, learned to keep her reaction to herself, and so when she couldn't avoid sex, she had a "let's get this over with" attitude toward it. As Anna described it, she had an automatic "no" reaction to almost any sexually intimate contact Brian directed at her. During lovemaking she did not like her breasts or buttocks to be touched. Her neck was ticklish, as were her thighs and feet. It was no wonder that sex was not very exciting for either Anna or Brian. Once Anna did the Parallel-Universe exercise, she saw sex in a different light. It did not have to be something you do for someone else. It could be something that would be good for her. Anna's reaction changed—when Brian initiated sex, she thought, "Why not?" Rarely could she come up with a good reason. Sometimes when they were lying in bed together or when they went on vacation together, Anna asked herself the same question: "Why not have sex?" She did not experience the powerful, lustful excitement that she had when she was pursuing Brian, but it was the first warming of her sexual feelings she had experienced in years. During lovemaking that same "Why not?" question surfaced when Brian touched her. Anna and Brian began to have satisfying sex again, and Anna often found that her physical desire for sex got ignited as she became aroused.

Remember that sexual desire is not something you feel only prior to sex. It is your wish, your motivation, and your physical urge to engage in sex that continues throughout the sexual encounter. In this way your desire drives behavior that increases your arousal, which in turn increases your desire—the desire-arousal feedback loop.

Expanding Our Definition of Desire

So now that you have some of your own motivation to work on your sexual desire (rather than doing it just for him), it is time to contemplate your next move. If you are serious about wanting to have sexual desire, then you need to stop engaging in obligatory sex, which reinforces old notions that sex is not for your enjoyment or benefit. You may believe that this means no more sex. On the contrary, you are expanding your definition of when sex is good for you. The old definition may only have included times when you already felt turned on. Most of us know that this should not be the only criterion. Being physically turned on does not necessarily mean that sex will be good for you. Emotional needs and physical safety have to be considered as well. If we all lived for the moment and had sex simply when we felt turned on to someone, there would be a higher incidence of STDs, pregnancies, coercive sex, broken hearts, and infidelities. Our decisions about whether and when to have sex have always included factors other than physical lust. To help clarify your decision-making process, consider the following three conditions as prerequisites for having sex:

1. I am arousable (open to being aroused).
2. I am feeling aroused.
3. I am interested in arousing my partner.

This last condition may have you puzzled, because it appears similar to having obligatory sex. But instead of being motivated to give your partner sex to placate him, you are motivated by a real desire to bring him pleasure. Under this condition sex will still be something that you do *with* him, not *for* him. While bringing him pleasure may please you or make you feel closer to him or feel sexy, it should not be the sole motivating factor all or even much of the time. Sometimes, on its own, the desire to turn your partner on can be fun, and in combination with either of the first two conditions, it can really improve the quality of your lovemaking.

If you wait to have feelings of sexual arousal before initiating or agreeing to sex, you may wait a long while. Remember that sexual desire is not just a physical sensation. It is also a willingness and a wish to have sex. Sometimes, if we linger over our wish and anticipate what might come to pass, we will begin to feel aroused. It may be a strong sensation; it may be a mild stirring. There may be no physical sensation at all to speak of.

It is well known that as they age, men need physical stimulation to get aroused. This is also true for women. So we'll run into trouble if we equate arousal with desire and despair when our imaginations and our partner's sexual invitations no longer stir us physically as often as they used to. As long as we can anticipate that sex will be an enjoyable and intimate experience, it will be something we will want. And as long as it is an intimate and enjoyable experience, our physical desire will be sparked. In Chapter 8 we will look at ways that we can keep our imaginations and our sexuality alive and vibrant, making those initial physical stirrings of desire more accessible to us.

Having sex only when you want to interrupts the negative-feedback loop you were previously in and replaces it with a healthier alternative—a cycle of sexual satisfaction. As the diagram below demonstrates, having sex when you desire it and believe that it is good for you will make it much more likely that you will put effort and energy into it. This in turn reinforces the notion that sex is good and pleasurable for you.

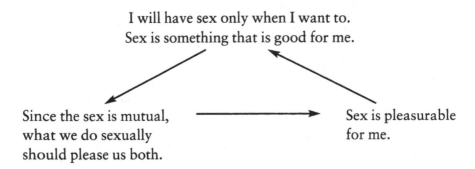

I will have sex only when I want to.
Sex is something that is good for me.

Since the sex is mutual, what we do sexually should please us both.

Sex is pleasurable for me.

Women who have kept their sexual desire and passion alive and well for an extended period of time have done so by making sure that sex was good, enjoyable, and fun for them. It was not something they did just to please the man in their life. This shouldn't sound selfish to you. Sex is the most pleasurable when it is a mutually enjoyable experience with each partner taking responsibility for his or her own passion. This is what keeps passion alive.

6

When Is Sex Right for You?

Longing springs from one's own nature
But there are ways to make it grow.
When intelligence has washed away anxiety,
Longing becomes unwavering and undying.

THE KAMASUTRA

Faking orgasms, having sex based on what you think will please your partner, and other similarly "unselfish" behaviors take you further and further from your own passion and desire. Do you think your passion is gone? Think again. Remember, sexual desire is not something that just jumps out of the blue, at least not once you have passed adolescence. Your sexual interest and desire will be sparked by the right conditions or circumstances. This chapter will help you get in touch with those conditions that will ignite your sexual desire, no matter how deeply buried it might be. Remember that you are trying to connect with your passion and not someone else's definition of it. Remember also that the circumstances under which you feel desire may be unique to you and may not be those that work for other women.

Liz had come to realize that her husband's curt and controlling behavior at home had killed her sexual desire for him. She knew that her lack of desire was not a physical problem, because she found herself fantasizing about other men. Liz loved her husband and wanted her marriage to work. She knew she needed to rekindle the passion she had once felt for Vince, but she did not know how to do this. In therapy Liz talked about the times that she had felt sexual desire for her husband, both in the recent and the remote past. At my encouragement Liz also talked about what had sexually interested her with other partners at other times in her life. Liz recalled that the last time she felt some stirrings of sexual interest in her husband was when Vince had purchased an antique rocking chair to surprise her. Many of the times that Liz recalled feeling desire for Vince were when he bought her something. The thought that she was materialistic depressed Liz. However, when she broadened the scope of her investigation, she found that with past partners and with Vince, she had felt the most desire when they had done something thoughtful for her. The feeling behind the thoughtful gestures was Liz's sense that she was loved and valued. Recently Vince had tried to show Liz that he cared about her by buying her gifts, but Liz realized that in order to feel sexual desire, she needed more than material things—she needed to feel that Vince valued her.

What follow are some writing exercises that will help you examine your sexual desire more closely. You may do all or just some of them. But understanding under what conditions your desire is likely to be sparked is of vital importance if you are serious about rekindling the passion in your relationship.

A Sexual Desire Time Line

When she looked back over her life, Liz realized something important about what she needed in order to feel sexual. You can do the same.

Think about the times that you have felt sexual. This may mean sexually responsive and enjoying sexual activity and/or sexually active and initiating sex. It may or may not have involved a partner. So think back over your life. When did you last feel sexual desire? Think back to the time before that and the time before that. Write down just a few words about what was going on in your life and in your relationship (if you had one) at the time. When you are done, look over the chronology and think about what these times had in common.

Sometimes when doing this exercise, women give up and say, "What's the point? I can't have what I want." Anna knew she felt passion when she was not in a committed relationship, but she had no intention of leaving her husband solely to be able to have good sex with relative strangers. When Anna examined how she *felt* when she was sexually passionate, she found more relevant insight. She discovered that she felt in control in these relationships. She knew what the men wanted, and she knew she could give it to them. She felt powerful. In addition to jotting down the times you felt desire, describe what was going on in your life at that time, highlighting the other emotions you were experiencing. Then look over your notes and see what patterns or similarities emerge.

Sexual Scripts

Whether we are aware of it or not, our behavior is often dictated by scripts. These are patterns of behavior that we follow, or believe we should follow, in particular situations. Scripts are especially helpful when we are confronting a new situation or a situation that makes us anxious. When invited to the home of someone I don't know very well, I follow a script. I dress nicely; I arrive on time; I bring a gift of food, wine, or flowers; and I offer to help my hosts (in the kitchen or cleaning up, for example). If this seems like common sense or common courtesy to you, then we share the same script. Scripts are dictated by our life experiences and also by our culture and the values and expectations of our families and the societies in which we live. An often-told story in my family was about the first time my father went to my maternal grandparents' home when he and my mother had just begun dating. My grandmother, ever the polite hostess, offered my father second helpings of dinner. My father politely refused. My grandmother offered again, and again my father politely refused. My father went home hungry that evening. You see, my grandmother was British, and in her culture asking twice if someone wanted second helpings was considered polite. Three times would have been pushy. My father had been raised in India, where you waited to be offered food at least three times in order to ensure that your host was sincere and could afford to provide you with more. As you can see, difficulties and misunderstandings arise when people are following different scripts.

Sexual scripts are the patterns of behavior that we follow, or believe we should follow, when we are engaging in any sexual interaction, from the initiation of sex to the proverbial cigarette afterward. Sexual problems can arise when lovers are following different sexual scripts or are following sexual scripts that are very different from the ideal script they have in mind.

Matthew and Beth consulted me with the complaint that Beth had low sexual desire and did not reach orgasm during sex. It was tempting to view Beth's disinterest as a reaction to the absence of orgasms. However, when I looked at the larger picture this couple presented, it became obvious that Matthew and Beth were following different sexual scripts.

Matthew, who desperately wanted his partner, Beth, to have an orgasm, was unconsciously following his own sexual script, with no thought that Beth might have other ideas about what constituted good sex. Matthew had come from a rather uptight, patriarchal family. He had suffered greatly because of his father's emotional abusiveness. In fact, his father had sold the family business to him for a great deal of money, only to open a competing concern a few months later, which ultimately put Mathew out of business and into debt.

Matthew was determined not to be like his father. He wanted to be generous and kind. This was his life script. This was why it was vitally important to him that the sexual pleasure be shared equally in his relationship with Beth. Magazines and talk shows discussed the importance of female orgasm. Matthew came to equate sexual pleasure with orgasm, and he was determined that Beth should have one.

Beth's sexual script was very different. She approached sex as she did most recreational pastimes. She was tentative and cautious and controlled. Beth had suffered what her family called a "nervous breakdown" when she had left home to go to college. It had devastated her family to have their daughter "fail" college and end up in a psychiatric hospital. Though this experience was now twenty years behind her, Beth still felt it important to keep her feelings muted and under control. She liked sex, she liked feeling close to Matthew, and she was troubled by his insistence on her orgasm. Beth had also been affected by the societal messages about orgasm. She was an avid reader; she subscribed to *Cosmopolitan* magazine and read steamy novels by authors like Harold Robbins. She became convinced that orgasms caused women to be wild and out of control. Beth was quite content never to be out of control again.

The next two exercises are designed to help you see what sexual script you have been following and how it differs from the script that you would like to follow. Remember, these exercises are designed to increase your knowledge and awareness of what you need in order to feel desire. Your script does not have to be realistic, in terms of your being able to actually act it out. It just has to be yours.

You're the Director

In this exercise first imagine that you are the director of a movie in which there is to be an explicit sex scene. This sex scene is your focus. Cast yourself as one of the main characters, and then choose the plot, the setting, the costumes, the relationship between the characters, the emotional tone and context—everything. Don't be limited by reality. This scene is yours; the purpose of the exercise is to represent your ideal sexual encounter. Write it down. When you are done, look over the script and ask yourself the following questions:

- What role did I play in the scene? Did I initiate things directly or indirectly? Was I seduced, cajoled, forced into it? When the sex got going, what role did I play? Was I active, passive, responsive?

- What role did my partner play? Was he active, passive, romantic, seductive, cavalier, distant? When the sex got going, what role did he play?

- What was the ambience or mood of the scene? Was it fun, playful, serious, romantic, passionate, safe, calm, coercive, frightening?

- What was the relationship between the main characters? Were they in love, strangers, best friends, old acquaintances, married? Imagine what came before they had sex and what happened afterward. Was there an argument? Were there kind gestures, familiar routines? Adventure? Danger? Love?

- How did I feel while the sex was occurring: aroused, dispassionate, loving, scared, safe, calm, excited? How did my partner feel?

- If there were others involved in my ideal sex scene, what was the nature of their involvement and why were they there? If there were others watching, what were their reactions? If others were participating, how did this affect me?

- What does my scene tell me about the conditions I need in order to be interested in sex? Are these conditions present in my current relationship? If not, how can I implement them?

Jennifer's script work provides a good illustration of the Director exercise.

> Jennifer imagined that she and Bill were having a romantic evening at home. He had planned everything—the dinner, the elegant table, the candlelight, and the wine. She was wearing an evening dress, and he was in a tuxedo. They ate dinner and talked about their intimate feelings. After dinner they slow-danced in their bare feet on the carpet. Then Jennifer imagined that Bill would lead her into the bedroom and they would make

love. She would be as active and involved as he was, but she saw everything happening in slow motion. Afterward they would lie in each other's arms and talk.

At first glance this script seems rather traditional, perhaps something borrowed from a romance novel. Jennifer's script, like many women's, is strongly influenced by the societal norms and values with which she was raised. But while societal norms may dictate the costumes and setting, Jennifer's script is otherwise quite revealing. The essential features of this script include the careful planning and detail, the fact that Bill takes care of everything, and the fact that the lovemaking happens in slow motion. Jennifer is often very stressed and feels as if sex competes with her stronger need to sleep. She often does not feel aroused, at least until she and Bill are already having sex. But in this scenario Jennifer has all the time in the world, to slow-dance, talk, and make love in slow motion. She is not tired. All the preparations have been made by Bill. Jennifer does not have to do a thing, until they are in bed, and then she wants to. In these relaxed conditions, Jennifer is convinced that she would have desire. However, the reality of her life—a full-time job, a young child, and all the stresses of modern living—makes such a scenario seem an unrealistic fantasy to Jennifer. Not so. Reducing her fantasy to the essential elements, we find the following necessary conditions for Jennifer's desire:

- She needs time. This means setting aside time to make love and not leave sex till the moment when she falls into bed exhausted.

- She needs some intimate involvement to precede sex, like some time talking or perhaps another shared activity.

- She needs Bill to take charge to see that numbers one and two above happen.

- She needs sex to proceed more slowly.

Jennifer's third condition is one that is often mentioned by women who are leading busy and stressful lives. They would love for their husband or partner to make the reservations, arrange for the baby-sitter, and let them relax and feel cared for. Condition number four is a very common one for many women, but it is especially relevant for women with low desire. Remember that often desire is not sparked until there is some arousal. If we want to ignite the feedback loop of arousal $\longrightarrow$ desire $\longrightarrow$ more arousal $\longrightarrow$ more desire, we need to take our time. If we don't have desire, we don't want our genitals to be touched or grabbed. When we have desire, the touching, stroking, and caressing of all parts of our bodies certainly feel more welcome.

Marissa, who had been date-raped, came to believe that her sexual desire was a dangerous feeling. She therefore followed a script that eliminated her desire from sexual activity. However, since she didn't have desire, she often felt that her husband was just grabbing at her. Doing the Director exercise was very helpful.

> In Marissa's ideal script, Frank had had a difficult day at work. He came home later than usual, after the children were in bed. Frank really needed to talk and unwind from his day. They sat in their hot tub and talked and relaxed for almost an hour. Marissa could tell that he felt better after talking with her. She felt needed and valued by him. She felt close to Frank and wanted to have sex with him. She could tell that he wanted to have sex with her, too. When they made love, she was responsive to his caresses.

Looking at the essential features of Marissa's script, we see that it was important to her that she felt that Frank valued talking to her and spending time with her apart from sex. As was the case with Jennifer, Marissa needed sex to proceed slowly in order for her to feel comfortable being touched. So the essential elements of Marissa's script were these:

- She needs some intimate involvement to precede sex.
- She needs to feel valued by Frank for more than sex.
- She needs to experience some sexual desire before Frank begins to caress her.
- She does not like to be surprised. She needs to know that sex is likely to happen.

When you do this exercise, you may find some elements that are different and some that are the same as Jennifer's and Marissa's. Many women are more interested in having sex when it is preceded by some other intimate activity. However, in our busy lives, this is often difficult to ensure. When Jennifer got around to implementing her script, she found that slowing sex down, rather than speeding it up to "get it over with," helped her interest, her desire, and her arousal. The intimate activity that she felt needed to precede sex was often accomplished during sex. She and Bill often laughed and talked before, during, and especially after lovemaking.

Slowing down and allowing for some time to have intimate contact during sex also helps deal with another difficulty. While women often feel more interested in sex after some intimate contact such as talking, men often find it easier to get their intimate contact from sex, or they are more willing to accept intimate contact after sex. At no time is this more apparent than after an argument. Men often make up by initiating sex, whereas women want to resolve the disagreement by talking first. Slowing down and incorporating more intimacy into sex, such as talking and laughing, can bridge this difference.

The importance of knowing what inspires passion and what defeats it cannot be overemphasized. Don't get caught trying to follow someone else's idea of passion. Follow your own script. The danger of following someone else's script is nicely illustrated by the misunderstanding that existed between Marissa and Frank.

Before Marissa came to therapy, she and Frank had made numerous attempts to improve the passion in their relationship. At no time did the pressure on Marissa feel greater than when a special occasion arose. Birthdays and anniversaries were difficult for Marissa, because she knew that her husband would want to have sex. She wanted to make him happy, and so they both fell back on a sexual script that they believed was the "right" script.

Their tenth anniversary provides an excellent example of the trouble Frank and Marissa encountered each time they followed this script. Frank made a reservation at a charming bed-and-breakfast in a neighboring town for the weekend closest to their anniversary. They had dinner reservations at a four-star restaurant for Saturday night, and Frank's sister was watching the children. It sounded perfect. All Frank asked of Marissa was that she wear a low-cut dress to dinner. This, he thought, would set the mood for a sexy and romantic evening.

Marissa complied, despite her misgivings. Marissa was very self-conscious about the size of her breasts. She felt that they were too large for low-cut outfits, and, far from feeling sexy, she felt like a slut. This, of course, was a passion killer for Marissa. She felt that all her husband wanted was sex, that all he would be doing through dinner was looking at her chest and going through the motions of conversation just to finally get her into bed. This was reminiscent of the date rape those twenty years ago. And, as you may recall, these conditions were the opposite of Marissa's conditions for experiencing desire. She needed to feel that Frank valued her and enjoyed her company. Each time Frank did something to try to make Marissa feel sexy, it usually backfired.

Once Marissa discovered her own conditions for feeling sexual, she was able to choose clothing that made her feel sexy but not sluttish. And despite Frank's expressed desire over their ten-year marriage for her to wear low-cut clothing, he never once complained. Months after their sex life had improved, Frank told Marissa that his suggestion that she wear low-cut dresses was meant to help spark their flagging relationship. Now that they had the spark, her clothing was not an issue.

You're the Critic—the Movie Critique Exercise

Because some women believe they lack imagination to create their own script, doing a movie critique is a good substitute for the Director exercise. If you have done the Director exercise, critiquing a sex scene in a movie can provide additional information and clarity as to what excites your passion.

Pick one or several movies that contain at least one sex scene you found erotic. The movie need not be X-rated; the sex does not have to be as explicit as it is in pornography. Indeed, many women who have used or tried to use pornography to jump-start their desire-arousal feedback loop are sorely disappointed. Often they find that the movies are turnoffs, because there is no plot, no character development, and an overemphasis on large penises and grateful, willing-to-do-anything women. Those women who do enjoy watching explicit movies most often do so with a partner with whom they have a good relationship (sexual and otherwise). They take the movies for what they are and are not expecting to see Academy Award material.

For the purposes of this exercise, think back to the movies that you really liked and the sex scene(s) in them. Choose a sex scene from one movie, and write down your answers to the following questions:

• Which character do I most identify with, and why?
• What do I find attractive about the other person in the scene?
• What is the relationship between the lovers, and what do I find compelling about it?
• What happens during the scene that I find erotic, interesting, or a turn-on, and what happens that turns me off?

We can learn a lot by paying attention to our tastes in books, movies, and television. Anna was able to get some insight into her conditions for desire by doing the Movie Critique exercise.

The movie Anna used was her favorite, *Out of Africa.* Not surprisingly, Anna had chosen a film in which the heroine is an independent woman who falls in love with a man who is always flying off and leaving. Anna felt upset when she recognized this pattern. She feared that this meant she was doomed to feel desire only in the pursuit of an unavailable man.

However, when Anna looked at the relationship between the characters, when she noticed how they interacted when they were together, she gained some new insight. She recalled that the characters shared a love of music and books and the beauty of Africa. The seduction was often verbal, and the sexual relationship seemed to flow from that. Anna identified with the independent spirit of the female lead, played by Meryl Streep. She was intrigued that this woman was so open about her desires and tried hard to get what she wanted. The turnoff for Anna was that the male lead, played by Robert Redford, seemed to be in complete and sole control of his comings and goings. Anna knew that that sort of arrangement would never work for her.

The necessary conditions for Anna's desire included these:

- She needs a sense of her own independence or autonomy.
- She needs a shared experience prior to sex.
- She needs the knowledge that she has some control within the relationship.

You Get Top Billing—Be the Star in the Scene

A follow-up to the Movie Critique exercise is to see what it would take to put yourself and your partner in the scene. The Movie Critique exercise will give you a sense of what qualities you find attractive in lovers, what an appealing dynamic is in the relationship between lovers, and what it is about the quality of the sexual relationship that is appealing. You need to think about what it would take to implement these conditions in your life. Put your partner and yourself in the scene, and write down your answers to the following questions:

- What will it take for me to have the qualities I admire in the heroine?
- Does my partner have the qualities I admire in the hero? If not, what are his admirable qualities?
- How can my partner and I relate in a way similar to what I found sexy in the movie?
- What are the sexual activities, or what is the quality of the sexual activities, that I would like to have in my sexual relationship?

Anna's answers helped her put her relationship into a better perspective.

Anna admired the heroine's independence and believed that she shared this characteristic. However, while the movie heroine's independence allowed her to share her thoughts and feelings with her lover, Anna recognized that her own independence precluded such intimate sharing. She rarely told Brian anything that happened in her day, let alone her thoughts and ideas. What Anna found attractive in the movie hero was that he was smart, independent, and an attentive lover. He seemed really interested in his lover's life. Although Anna recognized that Brian was a smart man, she felt that he was not a good listener, and she never felt as though he was interested in her life. Anna found the talking and the mutual interest and admiration in the movie lovers very compelling. She had to guess at a lot of what occurred sexually between them, because the movie left most of that to the imagination. Anna believed that the lovemaking would be slow, nonverbal, and focused on the woman's pleasure. As a result of the exercise, Anna made the following resolutions:

- To talk more with Brian and let him know what was going on in her life and in her mind. She recognized that she could not fault him for being disinterested when she never told him anything remotely interesting.

- To focus on Brian's positive qualities and let him know that she admired those characteristics. Anna did think that her husband was smart, that he was a good provider for her, and that he let her run her own life. He was a fairly liberated man.

- To interpret his sexual desire as interest in her instead of as neediness on his part. After all, the heroine in the movie didn't think Robert Redford was pathetic for wanting to have sex with her, so why should Anna feel that? She recognized that seeing her husband's sexual desire as needy was also a way of putting herself down.

- To slow down when having sex and to communicate nonverbally during sex.

Make a list of your resolutions or your plan of action after completing these exercises. Commit the plan to paper, and keep it where you will see it often enough to refresh your mind. Anna used hers as a bookmark.

How Can I Change If He Won't?

It's common for a woman to believe that her partner needs to change in order for her to feel desire. We give men tremendous power and burdensome responsibility for making sex good. Again, this is an old script pattern. While it is unlikely that you are solely responsible for your lack of passion, you can make the changes necessary for passion to ignite. Institute change unilaterally. You can, after all, change your own behavior and attitudes. Your partner's behavior will necessarily have to change in response. It really does take two to tango, and if you've switched to the fox trot, your partner will have to do some fancy footwork to keep dancing with you.

Don't panic if you think your script is vastly different from your partner's. You are not going to force him into anything. You are simply bringing your ideas about sex to the table or, perhaps more appropriately, to the bed. Scripts are flexible, and as long as your basic conditions are met, you may find that the costumes, the timing, and even the activities can and will vary.

Change Back

Taking on the responsibility for change does not imply that the problems are solely yours. Rather, it is the only perspective that will move you out of the passion-defeating mode you are currently in. Change is not likely to be instantaneous. Your partner is at least accustomed to the status quo. He may have his own reasons it works for him, despite the fact that he is unhappy with the lack of sexual passion on your part. Many men are comfortable with the relationship the way it is. They just want their partners to "fix" themselves so that sex occurs more often and more passionately. Harriet Lerner in *The Dance of*

Anger[1] describes what often happens when one person in a couple changes. Following the change there is a strong "change back" message from the partner. Brian's change-back message to Anna was delivered in the form of his failing to remember things she told him when she began to share her thoughts and feelings with him. In essence he was telling her that it was useless to talk. Anna did indeed get that message, but she persevered. She kept talking to Brian, and finally the change was incorporated into the relationship. Brian did enjoy having Anna talk to him, but his knee-jerk reaction was to tell her to go back to the way he was used to. Change, even for the better, is often upsetting. So if you take responsibility for instituting the conditions you need in order to feel sexual desire, you may get the change-back reaction. If you stay on course with your change, the relationship and your partner will accommodate.

A Word about Sexual Fantasies

Sexual fantasies can help put you in an erotic mood during or outside of sex with your partner. Examining your sexual fantasies can also help to determine what conditions you require in order to feel desire. However, in analyzing fantasies you run the risk of causing them to lose their appeal. This is why I recommend that you do the exercises and leave off dissecting your sexual fantasies. In fact, to enhance your feelings of desire, it is helpful to indulge the fantasy, to allow yourself time to have sexual daydreams. Again, this helps put you in an erotic mood and helps keep you there. Have no fear if your sexual fantasies are unusual or involve people and activities you would never want to be involved with in your real life. Fantasies are just that. They are a way for you to play in your mind, and they do not indicate that the imagined activities are what you really crave. The same is true of the sexual scenarios you came up with in the earlier exercises. Taking your fantasies and the sexual exercises that you work on in this book literally is a mistake. Lynda's story helps to get this point across.

Lynda is a forty-seven-year-old woman who came to see me because she wanted to feel sexual desire and arousal again after a twenty-three-year drought. Lynda had had an active sex life as a college student but had married a rather staid older man who she felt would provide her a more stable life. She was not sexually attracted to him, and sex with him was very routine, quick, and focused on his pleasure. Lynda felt hopeless about changing the situation, but she wanted to feel sexual again, if only on her own. Lynda had never had an orgasm, and she wanted this to change. Her rather puritan upbringing had made her feel that women should not fantasize about sex. However, as part of her solo work on her sexuality, she agreed to try the Director exercise.

Her first sexual scenario was extremely distressing to her. Lynda imagined that she was invited to a "lady's luncheon," but once there she was forced to be a "sex slave" for the other women. Lynda was concerned that this meant that she was a lesbian and furthermore that she wanted to be sexually coerced. However, as Lynda learned in therapy, sexual fantasies should not be interpreted literally. Lynda was just getting in touch with her sexual feelings. Women are sexual and erotic beings, and it is not unusual for women to tune in to this aspect and fantasize about having sex with other women.

Lynda is heterosexual, and no, she did not want to be coerced into sex. Lynda had no concept of her own sexual desire and so had to imagine a sexual scenario in which her desire did not play a role; in her story she had to engage in the sexual activities demanded by her hostess. Over time Lynda's fantasies changed, although she periodically revisited this initial scenario.

Anyone with an imagination can have sexual fantasies. There are specific exercises in Chapter 8 to help spark and enhance your sexual imagination.

Lessons Learned

Some of the case examples used in this chapter highlight some very common and almost universal truths for women dealing with sexual desire problems. Because the lessons that many of my clients learned were so important to them in reclaiming their desire, I've summarized them for you below.

- *Timing is everything.* Many men and women have a sexual script that involves the bedroom and hence bedtime as the time for sex. In our busy lives, we usually end up in our beds when we are physically and mentally exhausted. This is not a good time to begin to have sex. If we are going to value our sexual relationships, we need to set aside time for them. Just as we would set aside time to exercise, go over our finances, and review our children's homework, we need to set aside time for intimate contact with our partners. Many people balk at the notion of scheduled sex, but how is that so different from sex at bedtime? If we thought dinner out with friends should be spontaneous, it would never or rarely happen. I recommend that you routinely set aside time for some intimate contact with your partner. This will provide the opportunity for sex but does not necessarily demand it. So go to bed fifteen minutes to a half hour earlier each night with your partner, and use that time to talk, rub backs, snuggle, or have sex.

- *Slow down.* Many women who have little or no desire for sex rush through it as though it were an unpleasant duty to fulfill. They do not allow themselves to experience arousal, and so the desire-arousal feedback loop never comes into play. If you are going to have sex, you should enjoy it. So slow down and allow yourself that luxury. If sex is not enjoyable, you will find help for this in subsequent chapters.

- *Have some intimate involvement before, during, or after sex.* Many women crave intimacy with their partner; in fact, the lack of emotional closeness in their relationships precludes their desire. Men may initiate sex as a way to get close, but if a woman feels that all her partner wants is sex, she will reject the advance. If you slow down during sex, the question of whether intimacy should come before or after sex becomes moot. Of course, as we will discuss in the chapter on communication, sex is not the time to discuss dental appointments or other routine business, but it is a perfect time to share your feelings, some laughs, and/or a lot of tenderness.

- *Foreplay takes all day.* A sexual relationship is not sexual just at specified times and places. All interactions from the time we wake up to the time we go to sleep can either enhance or inhibit our sexual feelings and our readiness or willingness to have sex. Sexual desire gets turned off by unresolved arguments, criticism, sharp words, impatience, and other emotionally disconnecting or hurtful behavior. The old adage "Never go to bed angry" is still true. If you want to have a good sex life and feel desire for your partner, you must resolve differences and treat each other well during the day. Often a phone call at work or a hug while the dishes are being washed will do more to spark desire than the most romantic gesture in bed. You don't have to wait for your partner to institute this practice. Take charge, and if your partner doesn't reciprocate, read the next chapter, where I'll discuss tools to help you tell him what you want.

Women's sexual desire needs to be inspired, it needs to be elicited, and sometimes it needs a little coaxing. Understanding what conditions inspire your desire will help you not only to regain passion but also to understand that your sexuality is alive and well and awaiting the right opportunity.

7

Getting Your Signals Straight: It's All about Communication

Everybody lies about sex. People lie during sex. If it weren't for lies, there'd be no sex.

JERRY SEINFELD

The message many women receive about sex is that it is not something to talk honestly about. Many women were raised in families where sex was simply not discussed. Sex education, whether it takes place at home or at school, is never about sex but only about menstruation, reproduction, and the hazards of intercourse (disease, unwanted pregnancy). Abstinence-only sex education is a contradiction in terms. "Our crudest and oldest fear about letting out too much information is that it will lead kids to 'try this out at home' as soon as they are able," writes Judith Levine, the author of *Harmful to Minors: The Perils of Protecting Children from Sex*.[1] Somehow girls are supposed to grow into sexually happy and satisfied women once they say "I do."

Most women report that they primarily learned about sex from their friends and boyfriends. One's peers are not necessarily a well-informed or unbiased source of sexual information. If a girl talks too much about sex, she is labeled a "slut" or a "ho." So even among friends, a girl must rein in her sexual interest. The belief that girls want love and will trade sex for love when they feel they have to perpetuates the stereotype that girls don't have sexual desire. Myths and misunderstandings abound. Boys want sex; girls want love. Girls need to be protected from those boys who will do anything to get sex. (And boys need to be protected from girls who will do anything for a wedding ring.) Girls are taught about sexual exploitation and date rape and sexual violence (all of which are real), but they aren't taught about their own sexual desire, sexual pleasure, and sexual curiosity (which are equally real). From an early age, girls are given the message that sexual desire belongs to boys and that they must get love from these boys before they give them sex. If this refrain sounds familiar, it should. The struggle that adolescent girls go through is the same one that many adult women also experience: Under what conditions, if any, can she or "should" she want to have sex? Can sexual desire exist apart from love? If women's language of sexual desire is indistinguishable from the language of love, is this a true reflection of how women feel or the result of intense social pressure?

If women feel conflicted about their sexual desire and have little practice expressing their sexual interests, then it should come as no surprise that sex is difficult to talk about. Men are also not conflict-free when it comes to sex, and so they bring their own issues to the table. As a frustrated flight attendant might say, "Everyone has baggage."

Getting Past the Blame Game

The situation gets more complicated still when there is conflict between two people regarding the frequency of sex or the level of desire. Consider the following argument that I have heard repeated in my office innumerable times.

He: "You never want to have sex anymore!"

She: "We had sex just last week."

He: "Oh, and I should be happy with that?"

She: "I'm not saying that, it's just—"

He: "Let's face it, you just don't want to have sex anymore."

In this argument he is angry and blaming, while she is on the defensive. Nothing gets accomplished. At the end of this argument, this couple is not likely to fall into bed, nor are they likely to be remotely interested in doing so. Arguments about sex or the lack of sex invariably create distance in a couple.

Taking an offensive position also will not result in closeness or mutual understanding. Consider this possibility:

He: "You never want to have sex anymore!"

She: "Well, if you treated me a little better and did a little more around here, maybe I would."

He: "What, a reward for good behavior? I'm not a trained seal. Why don't you admit it? You just don't want to have sex."

In this discussion the barbs could go back and forth until one or the other or both are fatally wounded. Again, neither partner is feeling particularly close, intimate, or sexual at the end.

Women will often wish that "he would understand, that he would not be so angry"—in other words, they wish their partner would change. You might as well wish to win the lottery. It could happen, but it's not a good idea to count on it. What you can consider doing is being less defensive. Here's what that discussion might look like:

He: "You never want to have sex anymore!"

She: "You know, you're right. I'm not really interested in sex."

He: "Oh? So that's just the way it is? And you expect me to be happy about this?"

She: "No, I'm not happy, either. I wonder what we could do about it."

You could admit that you have low sexual desire—you and 33 million other women. It is nothing to be ashamed about. Recall from previous chapters that a lack of desire signals a problem with balance in your life; it is not an indictment of you. If you move from a defensive position, you will find a meeting ground that will allow for problem solving.

Change Back

Even in our communications, we will get the change-back message. If you cease to accept the blame for infrequent or unsatisfying sex ("There's nothing wrong with me—there's a problem in our life or my life"), your partner may not immediately agree with your new perception of the problem. You will get the change-back message—change back to the problem's being you. You need to persevere through change-back messages before lasting change is incorporated into the relationship. Here's what such an argument might sound like:

He: "You never want to have sex anymore!"

She: "You know, you're right. I'm not really interested in sex."

He: "Oh? So that's just the way it is? And you expect me to be happy about this?"

She: "No, I'm not happy, either. I wonder what we could do about it."

He: "I've tried everything, and nothing works. Stop making excuses. You don't want to have sex, and until that changes, there's nothing I can do."

She: "I know you've tried a lot of things. I've been reading about sexual desire problems in women, and I think that if we change some things about our life, our sex life will improve."

He: "That's just one more excuse, one more hoop to jump through. It never used to be this difficult."

She: "Our lives never used to be so complicated. Things have changed. A lot of women experience this same problem.

I think it's worth trying something else to see what we can do."

He: "Well, what is it that you want to do?"

Bingo! Now they're ready to solve the problem.

Remember, it wounds your partner to feel that you do not desire him any longer. When people are wounded, they tend to strike back. It may be less stressful for your partner to believe that there is something wrong with you than that there is something undesirable about him. But the choices are not simply your fault or his. As you've learned, the more likely problem is that your life is out of balance, that the conditions that will inspire your desire are not present. In other words, the *two of you* have a problem. Remember, *you* are not the problem.

What Is This Fight Really About?

Often arguments are about who is right or wrong or who has the upper hand, rather than serving as ways to work things out. If you identified an imbalance in power as one source of your low desire, you should pay particular attention to power plays in your communication. There is no winning in these arguments. The only way to get resolution is to step outside the power play. Do not become so invested in being right (or proving him wrong) that you sacrifice the possibility of having a satisfying relationship. People listen more effectively when they are not invested in being right. When you listen, you can learn a lot.

Arguments can also be a way of distancing oneself, and they can provide an excellent excuse for refusing sex you really don't want. Michelle and Tony, who were introduced in Chapter 3, fell into a pattern of hostile communication before bed.

Michelle was often resentful because she felt that she had to do things Tony's way. She had to cook the foods he liked, listen to the music he liked, and generally conduct her life so he would approve. Michelle felt an obligation to have sex with Tony, and she resented that, too. So, invariably in the evenings, Michelle would become very grouchy. Minor things would irritate her. She would bang the dishes around in the kitchen, complain that the cupboards were poorly designed, and swear loudly if she bumped against a piece of furniture. In essence, she made herself an unattractive person. She thought, "I may have to do these things, but I don't have to like them." She communicated the message, "Stay away from me." Tony got the message. If he tried to get close to Michelle or if he made a sexual overture, she would complain about her workload and insinuate that Tony did not do enough around the house. Inevitably after these arguments, Tony and Michelle would go to bed barely speaking.

Whether the issues Michelle raised were valid was not the point. Starting arguments, even valid ones, can be an effective means of avoiding sex. You do need to discuss problems with your partner, but at opportune times and with the earnest intention of trying to resolve them. Bringing up issues simply as a way to put your partner off perpetuates the anger and the distance in the relationship.

Not Tonight, I Have a Headache

Michelle and Tony's story highlights a difficulty many women have: how does one say no to sex? Perhaps if women could say no straightforwardly, they wouldn't have to say no indirectly, through arguments, avoidance, or pretense. When a woman complains that she has a headache (when she doesn't), she is reinforcing the belief that there must be a reason to say no. It's as if she needs to justify her position. Saying "I don't want to right now" is not acceptable.

Judith Levine quotes a prominent sex educator in Atlanta as saying that the most pressing concern of eighth-grade girls was to learn how to say no to sex without hurting a boy's feelings.[2] Many if not all of the women in my practice have voiced the same concern: how can they say no to sex without hurting their partner's feelings? The question of the eighth-grade girls is still a concern for adult women. The answer is complicated.

Occasionally saying no to sex is different than usually saying no. In the context of a vibrant and active sex life, both partners can recognize that they may not have similar sexual desires at similar times. However, the situation changes dramatically when "no" is heard more often than not or when the sexual relationship is fraught with tension and disappointment. So, given that your sexual relationship is in some trouble, you may ask how you can say no to your partner without his feeling hurt, wounded, rejected, or upset. The short answer is, you can't. The question you can ask yourself is, "How can I feel okay saying no to my partner, even though he may feel hurt and rejected?"

The answer is that you must evaluate yourself based on your actions and not on outcomes you cannot control. All you can do is say no in a kind, loving, and direct way. If your partner's feelings are hurt, that was not your intention. If you were kind in your refusal, you can feel okay about yourself. Paradoxically, the better you feel about being able to say no, the more often you may feel like saying yes. Feeling that you have to have sex or else suffer through an argument or endure your partner's hurt is a sure passion killer.

In order to see how you can refuse your partner's sexual invitation, we first need to discuss the difference between the message and the metamessage.

Maybe That's What You Heard, But That's Not What I Said

The message is what is contained in the literal meaning of the words. The metamessage is the meaning we infer from the context, the tone of voice, the body language, and the timing of the remark. People react to the metamessage; the meaning we attribute to the spoken word is the one that triggers an emotional reaction. Saying "I'm tired" literally *means* that one is fatigued. But it can also *suggest* disinterest, boredom, and avoidance. What you hear will most often reflect your own state of mind rather than the speaker's intentions. So if sex is a problem in the relationship, "No, I'm too tired" may be heard as "I can't be bothered" or some other dismissive sentiment. The key to improving sexual communication lies in recognizing the metamessages you are sending and the metamessages you are reacting to.

So what you believe you are communicating and what your partner is reacting to may be different. If you are not honest with yourself or your partner about the reason you are saying no to sex, there is little chance that the situation will improve. When you are not interested in having sex with your partner because you are not feeling particularly close to him, but instead you tell him you have a headache, not only are you perpetuating distance in the relationship but you are giving little opportunity for your partner to get the message that the quality of the relationship is important to your sexual desire. You may think he should know that. Don't get stuck in what he should or should not know. Tell him. Then when you have a headache or simply do not feel like having sex, your partner will be able to take the refusal at face value.

The Excruciatingly Correct Way to Decline a Sexual Invitation

Communication experts will tell you that the way to respond to someone in a caring, empathic way is to mirror back to him or her the feeling you heard in the request. So with a sexual invitation you would say something like, "I know you want to be close and intimate with me, and I appreciate that. However, I am very tired and have to get up to walk the dog at six A.M., so I am sorry to say I cannot have sex with you tonight." But let's face it—no one talks that way in the real world. What you can do is say no directly and nicely. You can be clear that you are refusing sex and not rejecting your partner. This can be communicated verbally and physically (get physically close or stay close). You can even offer your partner other options. Remember, there are more ways to answer than with a yes or a no. Here are some examples.

- "Thank you. No."
- "No, thank you."
- Say no, with an explanation. ("I'm too tired/I'm not feeling very close to you/I'm still angry/I'm just not in the mood. . . .")
- Use "I" statements, not blaming "you" statements. Avoid saying things like, "No, you've been rude and selfish all day." The refusal sounds like a punishment for bad behavior. It is more effective to say, "No, I don't feel very close to you right now, and I need to feel loved to feel like having sex."
- "I don't want to have sex, but I am interested in holding you/being held by you/holding you while you masturbate/having oral sex with you." Add the option only if you are truly interested.
- Be open to negotiation, but be prepared to stick to your original "no" if the counteroffers do not interest you. If you say, "No, I don't feel like having sex tonight," your partner may counter with, "Well, how about a quickie?" or "Do you mind if I masturbate?"

Many women use nonverbal communication to let their partner know that they are not interested in sex. They become physically distant and withdrawn. One man described feeling "a chill in the air" when his girlfriend did not want to have sex. But the message that gets communicated when we physically distance ourselves is, "I don't want to have anything to do with you right now." That may or may not be true. If it's not, there is really nothing wrong with communicating love, acceptance, and affection by being physically close while at the same time saying no to sex. The problem for many women is twofold: they worry about being a tease or leading their partner on, and they are uncomfortable saying no verbally. As you become more comfortable saying no to sex, and as sex becomes less of a contentious issue, it will be easier to maintain some physical affection and intimacy while still saying you don't want to have sex. While some men also distance themselves physically when their sexual overture is refused, most men like being cuddled up to even if the answer is no. What they don't like are confusing messages. So be clear: "I'm not interested in sex, but I still want to sleep spooned with you."

Never Having to Say You're Sorry

You do not need to apologize for your lack of desire. An apology puts you in a one-down position with your lover; it suggests that you are at fault. This may not be the message you intend to convey when you say, "I'm sorry, I don't want to have sex tonight," but it may be what your partner hears. The linguist Deborah Tannen[3] points out a gender difference in the meaning attributed to the phrase "I'm sorry." Women often say "I'm sorry" to express sympathy and concern, not to apologize. Men don't often say "I'm sorry," because they do not want to be put in a one-down position. To many men "I'm sorry" means an apology. It means "I was at fault." So when you say, "I'm sorry I don't want to have sex tonight," your partner might hear, "I don't want to have sex tonight, and it is wrong for me to feel that way." Your partner might also get the message that it is your fault that you do not want to have sex, but you may know that the reason for your not wanting to is that you've been up since six in the morning packing lunches for school, making breakfast, throwing in a wash, and getting to work on time. So if you want to express caring and make a connection to your partner despite not wanting to have sex, it is better to avoid saying "I'm sorry." You can express the connection physically, by snuggling close and kissing. You can express the caring in your tone of voice. And you can simply say any one of the things suggested above.

You Don't Love Me. You Just Want Sex!

How you respond to your partner's sexual advance depends on the metamessage you infer. Many women with low desire believe that their partner's sexual desire is selfish and is motivated solely by a desire to "get some." If you have little interest in sex, your partner's desire will seem out of context, inappropriate, and disconnecting. It may not feel like a gesture of love. The chances that you will feel like rejecting such an advance (whether you do or not) are high. The chances that you will feel turned on by such an invitation are low.

Take a few moments to think about the metamessage you get from your partner's sexual interest in you. Here's a list of some possibilities. Check all that you think apply to your situation.

☐ He's always horny.

☐ He thinks he can just jump into bed with me and I won't remember how badly he treated me all day.

☐ He has no consideration for the fact that I am tired/disinterested.

☐ He is so needy.

☐ He has too much testosterone.

☐ He needs to prove his masculinity.

☐ He is trying to make up to me. But this is not the way.

☐ He thinks he is such a great lover.

☐ Oh, great. He knows I don't get much pleasure from this, and yet his ego makes him keep trying.

☐ He thinks I should take care of his needs.

☐ Other _____.

Obviously these are downright negative interpretations of sexual overtures. Men generally aren't trying to send these messages, and no one would feel sexually inspired by them. Consider the possibility that you are misinterpreting the message. Consider everything you know about your partner. Certainly he has his flaws, as we all do. If you believe he cares about you, then get a different perspective on the situation. Step back so that you broaden the context in which you are judging the meaning of the sexual invitation and reevaluate the metamessage. Here's a list of some new possibilities. These are based on statements men have actually made regarding their sexual intentions.

☐ He really feels close to me when we have sex. When he initiates, that's what he wants, the closeness.

☐ He loves to make me feel good sexually. It's a way he has of showing me he loves me.

☐ He finds me attractive and desirable. I turn him on.

❏ He wants to make up to me for the things that happened during the day.

❏ Sex is fun. He wants to have fun with me.

❏ He knows that sex makes me feel closer to him. He wants me closer to him.

❏ He loves sex. He wants to share that with me.

❏ Other _____.

Try some of these out. Consider them as possibilities, or come up with some positive meanings to ascribe to your partner's sexual interest. After all, if he were so terrible and selfish, you would not want to stay with him. The next time your partner reaches for you sexually, consider a positive motivation. Your reaction will change. You may not want to say yes, but you will say no in a different way.

Let's look at what happened to Jennifer and Bill when they worked on the metamessages contained in their sexual interactions.

Jennifer was stressed out most of the time and felt that Bill's sexual advances were selfishly motivated and insensitive. She avoided Bill and sex. When Bill did reach out to touch her, Jennifer thought, "Oh, no, do I have to take care of Bill, too? I don't want to have sex, but if I say no, he will be mad. But if I say yes, I will be even more tired and stressed out." Jennifer felt there was no way to win in this situation. She knew if she refused sex, she would have Bill's angry feelings to contend with and she would feel guilty and bad about herself. On the other hand, if she agreed to sex, Jennifer would feel that she was simply giving in and giving up something of vital importance to herself. She would feel guilty and bad about herself. So most of the time Jennifer pretended to be asleep and avoided intimate contact with Bill. Bill was left feeling that Jennifer was too busy for him, that their relationship was a low priority for her, and that she no longer found him attractive or desirable.

When Jennifer evaluated Bill's sexual desire from a broad relationship perspective, she found that he was usually a loving man who cared about her needs as well as his own. Recalling her work in the Parallel-Universe exercise, Jennifer knew that if she felt desire, she would feel flattered by Bill's sexual interest in her. She would see his sexual interest as a desire to be connected to her. So now when Bill reaches out to stroke and touch Jennifer in a sexual way, she thinks, "He really wants to make a connection with me." She may or may not want to have sex with Bill, but she no longer has to avoid him. Jennifer even took advantage of the opportunity to address the reason behind her sexual disinterest. When she told Bill that she was too tired to have sex and wanted to sleep, she also told him, "I know I'm tired a lot. Maybe we can find a way to change things so I can have more energy for us."

You Are the Expert

In the next chapter, you will read about ways to get in touch with your own sexuality. For the purposes of this section on communication, it is important to emphasize the fact that you are the expert on you. You alone have access to all the information (thoughts, feelings, physical sensations, impulses, and so on) that will help you understand your sexuality. Too often we assume that men are the experts on sex, and when they tell us we should feel something and we don't, we wonder what is wrong with us. Many women who do not like breast stimulation, for example, have been told, "All women like their breasts to be touched. There must be something wrong with you." But women are not road maps, and going from point A to point B using the quickest, most direct route is not good lovemaking. Each woman is unique, with individual sexual preferences. This is why you need to be honest and authentic in your sexual communications. Being honest about what you like and don't like will help your partner be a better lover for you. When you are communicating your sexual preferences to your partner in an honest and straightforward manner, you are teaching him about pleasing you.

If Not Now—When?

Telling your partner when you do and don't want sex will help him understand what your conditions for desire are. It will also help your partner to know what helps get you in the mood for sex. Two common complaints that women have regarding the manner in which their partner initiates sex have to do with touching and timing.

Women often complain that how their partners initiate sex actually turns them off. For many women, being grabbed in especially sensitive areas (breasts, genitals, buttocks) is intrusive, annoying, and insulting. It reinforces the notion that she is a sex object. Most women have previous experience with being groped—in bars, on buses, or on the street—and therefore have a negative association to this type of touch. Now, this is not to say that playfully pinching, patting, squeezing, or touching certain body parts is always unacceptable; it's the context that is important. In the context of a vibrant and active sex life, such touch may be experienced as lighthearted teasing, a reminder of the intimacy of your relationship: "we can do this because we are lovers." In the context of a troubled sexual relationship, or when a woman has a history of unwanted touch, such "playfulness" backfires, and there is distance and anger and a feeling of being misunderstood by both parties.

Many of my clients have complained that their partner initiates sex at the most inopportune times, such as when they are going to work, late at night when they are tired, or five minutes before guests are due to arrive. Although it is counterintuitive, your partner may be anticipating rejection, and so he initiates sex at a time when rejection is most likely. That way when you say no, he can attribute the rejection to circumstances and not take it personally. If you say yes, it is a bonus. Then he can tell himself that you really must desire him, because you have thrown caution and good sense to the wind. If you feel that you must have sex with your partner when he wants it, you will be in a terrible bind in these situations and angry with the person you believe put you there. Remember though, that you do not have to satisfy your partner's every whim. You can enjoy feeling desired, but at the same time you can be clear that timing is important. If the timing reflects a knowledge of your schedule and a concern for you, sex is more likely to happen. If your boyfriend knows you are working late and has ordered Chinese food and put a bottle of wine in the refrigerator to chill, you are more likely to feel cared about and receptive to sex than if he waits until after you have fixed yourself something to eat and fall into bed exhausted.

Talking about Problems

Sex is difficult to talk about, and most people have little practice doing it. But it is better to talk about sex than not. With rare exceptions, sexual problems do not get better on their own. They get worse. When you are talking about sex, there are several things to keep in mind. Here is the most important rule: don't discuss sexual problems during sex. You may as well dump cold water on your partner during sex as you tell him that he ejaculates too quickly or that you have been faking orgasms.

The second most important rule is to initiate the discussion at an appropriate time, not during an argument but when the two of you are close and enjoying each other's company. Many women put off difficult discussions, and it's easy to do so. You don't want to ruin a good time, and you don't want to bring up such an intimate topic at a bad time. There will never be an ideal time to bring up the issue of sexual problems. Here are some helpful tips:

- Be proactive. Decide upon a time and then create the circumstances (time, space, mood, privacy) that will enable you to talk about the problem and maximize the chances that your partner will listen.

- You don't have to forewarn your partner. There is an old joke that the phrase men fear the most is "We have to talk." What your partner imagines you might want to say to him is likely to be far more drastic than what you actually say. Save him the stress.

- Keep the commitment you made to yourself to talk to your partner. Be direct. Say something like, "I want to talk to you about some sexual issues." You can follow this up with reassuring statements. "I want to talk about these issues because our sexual relationship is important to me."

- Use "I" statements. Instead of saying, "You don't turn me on the way you used to," you would say, "I don't get as excited about sex as I used to."

- Avoid the inclination to bring in outside experts such as friends, ex-boyfriends, and family members and their partners. Don't say, "I talked to my sister, and she thinks you're not very romantic, either. Her husband lights candles and draws her a bath when he wants to have sex." Such discussions almost always end in an argument.

- Feel free to make direct requests—for example, "I would really like it if you rubbed my back and kissed my neck."

- Accentuate the positive. Tell your partner what you do like. Reaffirm your interest in him.

Marissa wanted to make some changes in how she interacted with Frank during sex. What she said and did provides a good example of a woman's taking responsibility for talking about her sexual relationship.

Marissa knew how important it was for her to feel in control of her own sexual desire. During sex she maintained control over her desire by switching it off. She did not allow the desire-arousal feedback loop to get started. There were very few places on her body that Frank was allowed to touch. He had gotten the message and had long ago stopped trying. Once Marissa decided she wanted to get control over her desire by actively participating in sex, she had to communicate that to Frank. Her first attempts to tell him what she wanted during sex failed. Frank was confused by her sudden requests for different kinds of touch and complained that she was directing him "like a cop directs traffic."

So one evening when the children had gone to bed, Marissa invited Frank to join her in the hot tub. Then she told him how she felt frustrated about the limits she placed on their lovemaking. She told him that she wanted this to change, but she still wanted to be in control of her desire and her arousal. "Control" is a red-flag word to many people, and it may be especially so for men. Frank became angry and told Marissa that he did not want to be told what to do during sex. He told her that she needed to trust him, to be open to him, not to control him. The discussion turned into an argument, and Marissa went to bed in tears while Frank slept on the couch.

Marissa desperately wanted Frank to apologize and admit that he had overreacted. However, several days of stony silence passed between the two before Marissa decided to talk to Frank again and try to get her message across. This time Marissa did not use the word "control." Marissa began the discussion on a Saturday morning by bringing Frank a cup of coffee. She told him that she did love him and trust him. She knew that she had put restrictive limits on their sexual activities. She told Frank that it was her intention to be more open and trusting. She told him that she was going to try to communicate her desires to him during sex. Frank was able to receive this message without being defensive or angry.

Marissa did an excellent job of communicating to her husband. Although Frank liked to be in charge, it was Marissa who really took command of this situation. She was proactive and direct, and when she failed to get her point across on her first try, she tried again.

Mindy had a slightly different task. She wanted to talk to Calvin about changes she wanted him to make regarding sex. She was increasingly unhappy about Calvin's premature ejaculation. She had hoped that the problem would go away or that Calvin would fix it on his own. Mindy finally took responsibility for her own sexual pleasure and discussed her concerns with Calvin.

Mindy was quite fearful of talking to Calvin about her sexual dissatisfaction. However, the anger was building up inside her, and her unhappiness was "leaking" out in snide remarks, a short temper, and a disinterest in spending time with Calvin. Mindy knew she needed to address the problem. First she vented by expressing her anger, her disappointment, and her frustrations on paper. Then she ripped up what she'd written and went to talk to Calvin. She took Calvin's hand and looked at him, despite her inclination to look at her feet, the wall, the top of his head—anywhere except his eyes. She told him she loved him. She told him she wanted their sex life to be better, specifically that she wanted intercourse to last longer, because she really loved the feeling of having him inside her. When she looked at Calvin, she could see how difficult this was for him to hear. He could see how difficult this was for her to say. Mindy suggested that they go to see a therapist together, since they both had already tried to fix this problem on their own. Calvin was very reluctant and said he would think about it.

The next day Mindy looked in the Yellow Pages, made a few calls, and ultimately came to see me. Calvin had refused to accompany her, saying that he still felt this was something they could work out alone. He did not want to talk to a stranger about his "lousy sexual performance." So Mindy came on her own. Given that Calvin was not interested in starting therapy, I recommended they read a good book on male sexual problems. Mindy and Calvin read the book and did some of the exercises described in it. Then they both came to see me for several sessions, now that Calvin no longer felt so embarrassed and defensive. Mindy and Calvin found that their sex life vastly improved, not only in terms of Calvin's ejaculatory control but also in terms of their communication and their intimacy.

So Do You Want to . . . You Know . . . Nudge, Nudge, Wink, Wink?

Asking for sex is often a very difficult thing to do. Actually, it is something that few people do very well. The fact that we have no universally agreed-upon language for sex makes the task even more complicated. Do we call it "sex"? What about "making love"? "Fooling around"? Since we are not very practiced in talking honestly and openly about sex, we should expect some discomfort when we want to have it.

Opening up to another person and admitting that you have desires is not easy for women or for men. It is excruciating if the chances of rejection are high. Your partner may have told you he is tired of asking for sex and getting shot down. He may have told you that he will not ask anymore. While you might experience some temporary relief, you know that your partner still wants to have sex. Now you are in the awkward position of feeling that you must initiate when you don't really want to. In the short term, it always seems easier to avoid conflict and difficulties. In the long run, avoidance never pays off.

If the initiation of sex is now up to you, you may feel at a loss. So let's look at a few initiation dos and don'ts, to give you a better understanding of the complexities involved in making a sexual overture.

• Pay attention to your conditions for desire, and take responsibility for putting them in place. If you feel more sexually interested after sharing an activity with your partner, invite him to watch television with you, sit down and talk with him about your day, or join him in reading the Sunday paper.

• If the desire strikes you, act on it if you can. Don't wait until you have sorted the laundry or paid a few bills. Then you are acting as though your household chores or obligations are the priority.

• A sexual invitation has to be noticed in order to be effective. Some women who have successfully renewed their sexual desire find that their partner is so accustomed to their sexual disinterest that he fails to register a sexual advance when it is made. Make sure you are clearly expressing sexual interest. This is when it is helpful to have a shared language so you can say, "Do you want to make love/ fool around/have sex/lie down with me. . . ." If you are relying on nonverbal communication, you may need to clue your partner in, at least initially, until you are able to read each other's signals. So even though *you* may not like your genitals to be touched until later on in the process, most men don't mind having sex initiated by genital touching. It is a clear message of sexual interest and intent. Don't worry that sex will continue to be genitally focused. Once he has the message—and it shouldn't take long—you can remove your hand and caress other parts of his body.

• Accept the risk of rejection. Know that your partner may not be interested in sex when you are. He may say no. This is a clear message that, contrary to your belief, he is not always ready and willing to have sex. While this may be nice to know, your partner's refusal may hurt your feelings.

• Be open to negotiation. Just because you sent out the invitation, that does not mean you get to plan the whole party. You are inviting your partner to be sexual with you. He may want more sex or less sex or different sexual activities than you had in mind. The communication will need to continue. (More on that in the next chapter.)

• Be open to pleasure. If you have paid attention to your conditions for sex, you will not be initiating when you think *your partner* wants sex but when *you* will be more open to having sex. Don't wait for physical lust; know that the desire-arousal feedback loop may need time to kick in. Initiate sex with the expectation that you will get some sexual enjoyment out of it.

8

Sexercises for the Mind and Body

*Desire should be a longer word, multisyllabic.
There's such a distance in it, a wish for the
absent to be present.*

LORNA CROZIER

Consider sexual desire as a positive emotional state. Wanting, desiring, and anticipating pleasure and connection can be wonderful, whereas feeling obligated, duty-bound, and stressed is depressing and passion-defeating.

Even after you have understood the reason for you sexual disinterest, you may find it hard to rekindle the passion you once felt. Making changes in your life and in your relationship to correct what was out of balance may not automatically result in a resurgence of desire. You and your partner may find yourself stuck in patterns of behavior that perpetuate low desire. While women are inundated with information on how to become sexually desir*able* (just check out the headlines of the magazines the next time you're in line at the supermarket), how to become sexually desir*ous* can be a mystery.

In this chapter we will discuss how to embody sexual desire—that is, how to experience desire in your body. While the motivation for having sex or initiating sex may come from a desire for closeness and connection, it is important that at some point desire and arousal are physically experienced and expressed. Some of these exercises you will do on your own, and some are designed to be done with your partner. It is best if you do the solo exercises first, as the work you do on your own will be helpful when you begin to do the couples exercises.

Solo Exercises

Exercise enhances sexual desire and sexual pleasure, and it makes people feel generally sexier. Exercise makes sex better because it improves many of the bodily functions involved in sexual activity and desire. It increases blood flow, develops endurance, strengthens muscles, and builds muscle tone. Exercise also has psychological benefits that enhance sexual desire. Exercise is a great way to reduce stress, elevate mood, and increase self-esteem and self-confidence, all of which lead to better sex and heightened sexual desire. Men and women who exercise do not show the declines in sexual pleasure that accompany poor health otherwise associated with aging. Women who regularly exercise report that they are more easily aroused, achieve orgasm more often, feel more confident sexually, and have more frequent sex.[1]

Even if you are not convinced that exercise will help your sex life, it has health benefits that make it worth the effort. Books such as *Strong Women Stay Young*[2] make a compelling argument that exercise is essential for women who want to enjoy a long and happy life. It is never too late to start, and no amount is too little to do in the beginning. So as part of your plan to increase desire, include some regular physical exercise. It will be one more way that you make yourself a priority.

The best way to know if you are succeeding in your pursuit of desire is to keep track of your progress, no matter how minute. Consider keeping a diary in which to chart your daily progress. What did you do today to work on sexual desire? Did you feel any desire spontaneously? Which exercise did you do? Was it more difficult, easier, or more satisfying than the last time you tried? What did you learn about yourself and your lover? Take a few moments before sleeping or upon awakening to jot down your thoughts. At least once a week, look over what you have written and see how it has changed over time. Progress, no matter how slow, is rewarding and can keep you motivated.

Stimulating Your Sexual Imagination

In order to revive your desire physically, you will need to stimulate your mind. Your mind and body are connected, and if the spirit is not willing, neither will the flesh be. Sex needs to stop being an obligation, something you *should* be doing for someone else, and become exciting to you again. If you feel that you have little or no sexual imagination, don't worry. Your imagination may be suffering from lack of use. Here are some suggestions as to how to stimulate your sexual imagination:

• Go to your bookstore (or even browse online) and find some books on sex that appeal to you. Read them with a curious mind, asking, "Do people really do these things? I wonder what that would feel like? I'm going to have a fantasy about that. I think I'll try it!" Some reading suggestions can be found in the Resources section at the end of this book.

• Another boost to your sexual imagination can come, believe it or not, from shopping. And you don't even have to buy anything, unless you want to and can afford to. Go into a shop that sells beauty products and lotions. They almost always have samples that you can smell and try. Try massaging some lotions into your hands, and enjoy the sensuality of it. If you are adventurous, go into a sex shop and check out the products they have there. If you are timid about this, look online. You may find things that are humorous, sexy, or shocking, but your mind and your imagination will be exercised.

• Watch some erotic or pornographic movies. Go ahead—it could be fun. Watch the movie alone or with your partner.

• Read some sexy magazines alone or with your partner. Many women get turned on looking at *Playboy* or *Penthouse*. It is not because they want to have sex with women, but because they are tuning in to the erotic and sexual aspects of the pictures and stories.

• Look through some lingerie catalogs. If you feel so inclined, order something sexy for yourself or for your partner.

• When you see an attractive stranger, indulge in a little sexual fantasy.

Try to do something that sparks your sexual imagination every day. After a week or two, you may notice that you are having sexual thoughts spontaneously. This is the time to get your body in on the act.

Focused Breathing

Many women with low sexual desire have avoided sex and sexual feelings for quite some time. In order to restore sexual desire, it is important to focus in on these feelings. Recognizing the signs that you are aroused or sexually interested is extremely important. This exercise stresses breathing and meditation as tools to help you get in touch with or reawaken your sexual energy.

1. Sit comfortably, and place one hand on your chest, the other on your abdomen.

2. Relax your stomach muscles, and inhale deeply through your nostrils, completely filling your lungs from the bottom up. If you are doing this correctly, the hand on your chest should stay relatively still, while the hand on your abdomen will rise and fall with each breath.

3. Breathe in slowly to the count of five, then exhale slowly through your nose or mouth, also to the count of five.

Practice doing this focused breathing for several minutes each day, and use it during the day to relax, to alleviate stress, or to focus. Once you are able to do the focused breathing, you can add the following meditation to enhance sexual desire.

Sensual Meditation

1. Set aside thirty minutes of uninterrupted private time.
2. Lie down on your bed or relax in a comfortable armchair. If you are sitting, do not cross your legs.
3. Close your eyes, and do the focused breathing, described above.
4. After several deep breaths, begin to focus your attention on specific parts of your body one at a time. Start with your head, and work your way down, paying special attention to the sensual parts of your body. These will most likely include your lips, neck, breasts, abdomen, buttocks, inner thighs, and genitals.
5. As you direct your attention to each body part, try to relax the tension within it. Let a feeling of warmth inhabit your body as you focus on relaxing and releasing any tension that may be within that part of your body. Spend at least two minutes on each body part. It is important to continue the focused breathing.
6. When you begin to focus on your genitals, tense the muscles in that area, then release the tension. Do this several times while breathing and focusing in on the sensations you are experiencing. (To more specifically target the muscles around your genitals, try doing the Kegel exercises outlined next.)
7. Do this exercise at least once as directed above.
8. Add sexual fantasy the next time you do the exercise. So, in addition to focusing on a sense of warmth and relaxation, now incorporate a favorite sexual fantasy. If you do not have one, try imagining that your lover (or someone else) is kissing, touching, caressing, or stimulating that part of your body. Concentrate on the good feelings those thoughts inspire.

Do this exercise as often as you can. You can even do it before you go to sleep at night. Try to do it at least twice a week for about six weeks or until your desire returns.

Kegels

Kegel exercises, so named for the obstetrician who developed them, were initially designed to help women control incontinence following childbirth. The objective was to strengthen the musculature surrounding the urethra, which may have been weakened during delivery. However, Dr. Kegel's patients began reporting a welcome and surprising side effect of these exercises—enhanced sexual pleasure. Kegel exercises are now routinely prescribed by sex therapists to help women increase their sexual enjoyment, raise sexual awareness, and improve sexual functioning. Raising your sexual awareness will help you to experience and enhance feelings of sexual desire. Kegel exercises are easy to do.

1. Identify the muscle that you want to strengthen. This muscle is called the pubococcygeous muscle, or PC muscle. It surrounds the vaginal opening and the urethra. To identify the PC muscle, simply stop the flow of urine when you are using the toilet. Do not tense your thighs. You want to isolate and identify the movement of this single muscle.

2. Check that you have correctly identified the PC muscle. If you are unsure as to whether you are correctly identifying and isolating the PC muscle, there are two ways to check. First you can lie down on a bed with your clothing off from the waist down. Place a small mirror between your legs so that you can see your genitals. Tense and relax the PC muscle. You may be able to see movement as the muscle contracts. If you can't see movement, try inserting a finger into your vagina. You should feel some tightening around your finger as the muscle contracts.

3. Do the Kegels. Once you have identified this movement, practice it when you are not using the toilet. Simply contract the muscle, imagine that you are sucking water up into your vagina, and then bear down and relax the PC muscle. Imagine that you are expelling water or a tampon from your vagina. Repeat this ten times.

4. Then do slow Kegels. First contract or tense the PC muscle and hold the tension for a slow count of three. Then release or relax the PC muscle again to a slow count of three. Wait for a count of three, and then repeat ten times.

5. Next do quick Kegels, contracting and releasing the PC muscle in rapid succession. It should take a quick count of one to tense and

on the count of two release, on the count of three tense, on the count of four release. Do this four-count repetition ten times.

6. Repeat. Practice the Kegels for at least five minutes each day. Do at least one set of regular Kegels, one set of slow Kegels, and one set of quick Kegels. The beauty of the Kegel exercises is that they let you multitask. You can do them while ironing, watching television, reading a book, talking on the phone, or doing any number of other activities. No one will know but you.

It may take some time before you feel the effects of this exercise, but keep practicing. After a week or two, you should begin to feel some sexual arousal or interest when you do the Kegels. You may also notice increased sexual pleasure during sex with yourself or your partner.

Once you do the Kegels with relative ease and you are at least beginning to feel some sexual sensations, add sexual fantasy. During your five-minute daily Kegel routine, begin to think of something sexually arousing or appealing. Continue to fantasize while doing the Kegels.

Now add sex, alone or with your partner. You can do Kegel exercises during sex with yourself or your partner to enhance the sexual sensations. Try a few Kegels to help spur on your initial stirrings of arousal. Try some Kegels as you approach or experience orgasm. Some women find it especially pleasurable to tighten the PC muscles when they are having vaginal intercourse. They like the sensation as their vagina tightens around their partner's penis. Their partner usually finds it extremely pleasurable as well.

Self-Pleasuring

If your sexual desire has diminished, it is likely to have affected the sexual activities you do with your partner and on your own. Even if you have continued to masturbate, follow the steps outlined in this exercise to increase your sexual interest and awareness.

1. Know your conditions for solo sex. Think about what you need in order to feel comfortable masturbating. For many women this

eans privacy, either having the whole house or apartment to themselves or at least having the security of a locked door. Whatever your conditions are, note them and then make sure that you have them in place at least three times over the next ten days. You'll need at least thirty minutes with no distractions to do the self-pleasuring exercise. Unplug the phone, don't answer the door, and turn off the television.

2. Don't wait until you feel like masturbating to do this exercise. Do it when your conditions are in place. Set aside the time, and do the exercise whether you feel like doing it or not. You are trying to jump-start your sexual interest, not wait around hoping something will inspire you.

3. Get undressed or, if that feels too uncomfortable, wear loose and sexy clothing, such as a camisole or a nightgown.

4. Imagine the following scenario. You have awoken from a coma and are discovering your body and its responses to a variety of stimuli, as if for the first time. As you begin to touch your body, do so in a curious and appreciative manner. Start by being aware of the shape and texture of your body and your skin.

5. Caress your whole body and then begin to focus in on those parts that feel especially sensual or that help you get slightly turned on.

6. Visualize your desire building slowly. Imagine slowly ascending a long staircase. With each step your desire increases, but make sure that you rest and enjoy each step before proceeding to the next.

7. Stop on each stair, breathe deeply, and focus in on what you are feeling in your body and where.

8. Tease yourself. Allow your arousal to build, and then let it subside slightly. When you are nearing the top of the staircase (which for some women will mean orgasm), take a step or two back before going ahead again. Be aware of wanting to do more. Enjoy the feeling of wanting before you rush to satisfy it. This is desire.

9. Add a few Kegels while you are nearing climax to enhance your desire and pleasure.

10. Allow yourself to experience an orgasm. Really pay attention to what is going on in your body as you enjoy the sensations. As your orgasm subsides, imagine that you are sliding down the banister of

the staircase, and enjoy the thrill and physical sensations as your body returns to its resting state.

11. Climb the staircase again if you feel like it.

Exercises for You and Your Partner

When you are ready to do some of the exercises with your partner, it is important to discuss them with him first. Many women feel uncomfortable asking their partner to share the exercises. They feel silly or are convinced that their partner will not be interested. In my experience, while a woman's partner often initially balks at doing the exercises, once he has done a couple, he enjoys them and learns something from them. Don't be shy. Your partner should be gratified that you care enough about your sexual relationship to work on it.

Outercourse

Couples who have been together for a long time often get caught up in routine sex. They do the same or similar things in roughly the same order every time they make love. In order to improve sexual communication with your partner and add some variety to sex, try the following exercise. In this exercise, intercourse is not allowed. Eliminating this one activity changes the routine of sex. Once the routine is varied, you have to tune in to your partner and he to you to figure out what you would like to do next. Paying attention to what you *feel* like doing sexually is a way to enhance desire.

1. Discuss the exercise with your partner. Make sure you are clear that intercourse is not allowed. Make sure that your partner understands the purpose of the exercise and is in agreement to do this.

2. Ask your partner to be the rules enforcer. Since you are interested in exploring your desire, it is counterproductive to have to worry that your partner will violate the rules or forget about his agreement. Ask him to make sure that intercourse does not occur—that he does not attempt it, nor do you. You can add an incentive for

him: tell him he can be in charge of the remote control for the next week if he enforces the rules, but do not bargain for sex. Do not promise intercourse tomorrow in exchange for outercourse today, or you will revert to having obligatory sex once again.

3. Refer back to the conditions for sex you established in Chapter 6 and, with these conditions in mind, settle on a time to do the exercise with your partner. Set aside at least thirty minutes and no more than one hour. Make sure that you have privacy and are free from distractions such as telephones, television, and other interruptions.

4. During the exercise you and your partner will follow these communication rules: you are allowed to give only positive feedback. If you like something, express your appreciation *non*verbally. If you don't like something the other person is doing, express this verbally, using only positively worded messages. For example, if your partner is touching you too softly, you might say, "I really like it when you use more pressure in your touch," or "I prefer it when you caress me with your whole hand instead of your fingertips."

5. Spend at least five minutes after you have completed the exercise talking about it. Each of you should express a minimum of two things that you learned from doing this exercise. If you need clarification about something that occurred during your time together, ask about it. For example, one of you might say, "I always thought you liked it when I tickled your thigh," and the other might respond, "I do like it sometimes, but I just didn't feel like it today."

6. Do this exercise more than once. The more you do it, the more you will learn to tune in to your desire. Try to schedule this in at least three times this month.

7. After you have done this exercise at least three times, you can vary the rules. One variation is to include intercourse, but do not have it be the last thing you do. So the stipulation would be that your partner cannot ejaculate during intercourse. Another variation would be to extend sex beyond your partner's orgasm. Many couples believe that sex ends when the man ejaculates. Shattering this and other assumptions will make communication between the two of you essential. You will also learn how to have more variety and hopefully more fun during sex. Finally you can play a game between yourselves to see how many different ways you can satisfy each other sexually

before repeating any. Don't necessarily equate satisfaction with orgasm. When you do these exercises, focus on your feelings of fulfillment to help you determine when to stop a certain activity or change to a new one.

Mirroring

In this exercise you and your partner take turns mirroring the sensual and sexual movements of the other. The purpose is to focus your attention on your lover and, using only eye contact and body language, mirror his or her movements. You must give up your preconceived ideas of what the other person may or may not do in order to mirror effectively. This exercise improves nonverbal communication and helps you to teach your partner what turns you on. It also gives you an opportunity to learn how to really tune in to your partner's body language and to be a more sensitive lover.

1. Refer back to your conditions for sex and, with these conditions in mind, settle on a time to do this exercise with your partner. Set aside approximately one hour. Make sure that you have privacy and are free from distractions such as telephones, television, and other interruptions.

2. It is best if you are both completely undressed, but if that feels too uncomfortable, then wear underwear or light sleepwear.

3. Take turns being the leader and the mirror (the person mirroring the movements of the other). Using slow movements and sensual touch, the leader moves her body, touches her body, or touches her partner's body while he mirrors the movements. If she touches her body, he touches his in the same manner. If she touches his body, he touches hers in the same manner, with the same strokes and pressure. The leader touches her mirror's body in the places and manner that she would like him to touch her. If she likes light touch on her arms and kisses on her neck, this is what she does to her partner, and he does it back to her in the same manner. If he doesn't get it right the first time, the leader keeps repeating it until he does. After about twenty minutes, switch roles: the mirror becomes the leader, and the leader takes over as the mirror.

4. It does not really matter who goes first, although in my experience the man is usually more comfortable if his partner starts, but you can decide by coin toss or negotiation.

5. Do this exercise in several stages. When you first do the Mirroring exercise, divide your time as follows: For the first ten minutes, there is to be no touching of the breasts and genitals. The next five minutes can include breasts, and the last five minutes can include genitals. As you repeat the exercise, you can shorten the time spent on other body parts and focus more attention on breasts and genitals if you so desire.

6. Do not (and this is important) focus on sexually arousing the other person or bring him or her to orgasm. The purpose is for each of you to teach the other about your sexual preferences and to enhance nonverbal communication.

7. It is important not to have sex during or after this exercise. Otherwise all the sexual issues that are lurking in your relationship will infect the exercise as well.

8. After the exercise is over, you can talk about what you discovered or ask questions and get clarification on things you are still wondering about.

9. Repeat this exercise as often as you like. Try to do it at least three times before proceeding to the Mutual Pleasuring exercise.

Mutual Pleasuring

This exercise is a good follow-up to the Mirroring exercise and allows you to use what you have learned about arousing your partner and communicating with him. It also provides a good way to experience desire and then act on it.

1. Refer back to your conditions for sex and, with these conditions in mind, settle on a time to do this exercise with your partner. Set aside approximately forty-five minutes to one hour. Make sure that you have privacy and are free from distractions such as telephones, television, and other interruptions.

2. It is best if you are both completely undressed, but if that feels too uncomfortable, then wear underwear or light sleepwear.

3. You and your partner take turns being the giver and receiver of pleasure. Your partner is the giver first, and you are the receiver. After twenty minutes you switch roles.

4. The giver touches and caresses his partner with his hands, fingers, tongue, and body (and in later versions his penis) in places and in the manner he knows she likes (he has learned this from the previous exercises). The receiver passively receives this pleasure. As a receiver you do not reciprocate the touch but instead lie back and enjoy the pleasure your partner is bringing you. Allow your arousal and desire to build. The desire-arousal feedback loop should kick in. Let yourself simply enjoy the feeling.

5. When you are the giver, you caress your partner with your hands, fingers, tongue, and body (and in later versions your breasts if you should choose) in places and in the manner you know he likes. He passively receives this pleasure.

6. During the exercise you and your partner will follow the communication rules you used in the Outercourse exercise. You are allowed to give only positive feedback. If you like something, express your appreciation *non*verbally. If you don't like something the other person is doing, express this verbally, using only positively worded messages.

7. The first time you do this exercise, there is no touching of the breasts or genitals at all. The pleasure will be primarily sensual, not sexual. The second time you do this exercise, you may incorporate the breasts and genitals, but do not spend inordinate amounts of time on these areas. Make sure at least ten minutes are spent on nongenital touching. Low levels of sexual arousal should occur. The third time you do the exercise, you may each focus on those body areas that are the most pleasurable for your partner, resulting in higher levels of arousal and orgasm if you choose. It is important to do this exercise in stages, so that you can learn pleasuring touch and good communication first in low-pressure situations. You will also give yourself time to be comfortable with increasing levels of desire.

8. It is important not to engage in any other sexual activity during or after this exercise. Otherwise all the sexual issues that are lurking in your relationship will infect the exercise as well. Your partner may

indulge you in the course of doing the exercise, whereas he would not take it so well to be directed in sexual activity. Any reluctance you have to have sex will transfer to the exercise if you have sex during or immediately after. Once your sexual relationship is stronger, by all means incorporate this exercise or any of the others into your love-making.

Once you have done the exercises outlined in this chapter, do not go back to sex as usual. Remember what worked well for you in the exercises, what you liked, what made you feel desire, what turned you on. Apply the communication skills you learned from the exercises. Focus on your arousal to enhance desire and use the Kegel exercises to enhance your pleasure. By continuing to do these exercises and incorporating them into your sexual relationship, you will embody your sexual desire, be more comfortable with desire, and you will get the desire-arousal feedback loop working. Sex will become a mutual activity that you can look forward to again.

Sexual Attitudes

How you approach these exercises and, indeed, how you approach sex is vitally important in either inspiring or draining your passion. To maintain a positive outlook on sex, keep the following things in mind:

• *Slow down.* Do not rush through the exercises. Do not rush through sex. When you slow down, you can focus on your desire, your arousal, and your pleasure. You can give the desire-arousal feedback loop time to get going. Linger, enjoy, and experience the pleasure that can come from these exercises and from making a sexual connection with your partner. Focused breathing can help you slow down and tune in to your sexual self.

• *Be curious.* Curiosity about sexuality is a precursor to desire. It is an attitude that is open to possibility. Remaining curious will make it harder to get stuck in a routine sexual script, and it will be difficult for sexual boredom to take hold, now or in the future.

- *Be a sexual agent, not a sexual object.* Just doing the exercises in this chapter takes you out of the sexually passive role that your lack of desire has put you in. By implementing even some of the suggestions in this chapter, you are taking charge of your own sexuality. In and of itself, this should go a long way to improving your level of desire. Taking a more active stance in your sexual relationship also makes unnecessary some of the more covert maneuvers you may have engaged in to avoid sex. You have no chance of experiencing your own sexual desire when you are busy resisting someone else's.

- *Don't limit sex to the bedroom.* Be conscious of maintaining the connection that you are establishing by doing these exercises with your partner. Enjoy holding hands, exchanging loving glances, cuddling on the sofa, and kissing. These are many of the things you used to do before sex was an issue and many of the things that couples with active sex lives share.

Problems and Pitfalls

Many women with low desire will not feel like doing these exercises. This will be especially true if you have not done some of the earlier work on motivation suggested in Chapters 5 and 6. If you have skipped over some of the earlier work, go back and complete it now. If you have done the earlier work and are still having problems doing the exercises, look down the following list and see what issues may be surfacing for you.

- *Time.* As a mother of two, I certainly understand that getting thirty minutes or more of uninterrupted time is very difficult, and there are other things that you may need to accomplish in those precious minutes (such as cooking, eating, sleeping, paying the bills, doing paperwork, and talking to your partner). If you don't have time for the exercises, then you certainly don't have time to have great sex. The first thing you may need to work on is getting time. Some things you can consider include hiring a babysitter even when you are staying home, exchanging "play dates" or babysitting time with friends and neighbors, putting the children to bed earlier, getting a lock on your bedroom door and using it, and taking advantage of times when the children are occupied (what else are Saturday-morning cartoons for?).

• *General fears.* Some women get stuck at this stage because of a fear that if she doesn't control the frequency of sex, no one will. Often the fear is that her partner will want to have sex all the time, that she will be on a roller coaster with no brakes. While this fear is understandable, it is hardly logical. Unless you are partnered with a sex maniac, it is likely that your partner will be looking for a fulfilling relationship and will not be fixated on racking up notches on the proverbial belt. Nevertheless, the best way to counteract this fear is to be aware that you have the ability to say no to your partner. Go back to the chapter on communication and reread the section on how to say no to sex.

• *Communication problems.* If you haven't let your partner in on what you are doing, then you may be giving him a mixed or confusing message. Remember that your partner may be feeling insecure due to your lack of desire for him. He may see the fact that you are spending more time on your own and buying lingerie and lotions as a sign that you are interested in someone else. He might feel hurt and confused by tender touches that are not followed up on if he is not aware of what you are doing. Tell your partner what is going on.

• *Change-back messages from yourself.* More than ever, you are challenging the status quo of your relationship. You are taking charge of your sexuality. It may raise your anxiety to do this. If power and control and/or intimacy were imbalances you identified earlier, you may be telling yourself to change back to the status quo to reduce your own anxiety. If avoiding sex has been about avoiding intimacy, then your issues with intimacy will be reactivated with these exercises. The change-back message may come in many different guises. It may seem to you that this is too hard, that life wasn't really so bad before, that the exercises are silly or ineffective (before you have even tried them). Examine the statements you are making to yourself, and if they result in the conclusion to change back, you need to recognize this. Change-back messages will help you cope with anxiety through avoidance, but they will not help you make progress. Work through the change-back message, even if it makes you feel anxious. In other words, push yourself to do the exercises.

• *Change-back messages from him.* Especially if one of the imbalances you noted was in the area of power and control, the change-back message may come from your partner. He may be unhappy with the lack of sex, but he may like other parts of the status quo. Even if you have told him what you are doing, he may be less than supportive. Some men have mocked or belittled their partner's attempts to address the desire issue. For many men, having their wife or girlfriend need to *work* on desiring them makes them feel less than desirable. So your partner may poke fun at your attempts or otherwise subvert your efforts. Treat this as you would any other change-back message: stay the course.

• *Low sexual self-esteem.* It is not just perfect bodies that are erotic. They may be the most pleasing to look at, and the airbrushed centerfolds and the cover "girls" (and yes, most of them are girls or just barely adults!) have made us believe that sexiness is an appearance issue. But a few extra pounds, some wrinkles, and not-so-perfect proportions can be found on the bodies of the most ardent lovers. Your body is capable of receiving and giving pleasure, even if it is not a perfect 10. Treat it well. Pamper your body. This doesn't mean that you have to spend a lot of money. Mostly it means taking time. Moisturizing lotion from the drugstore, lovingly applied, can be as sensual as an expensive lotion from a world-class spa. Sexy is attitude. When you criticize and denigrate your body, you diminish that erotic potential. When you are thinking about your body and your appearance, ask yourself whether you are taking good care of yourself. Do those extra pounds mean that you are not eating well or not exercising—or are they just the way you are built? Are those creases around your eyes crow's-feet or laugh lines? It's all in how you look at it. As the population ages, if we are lucky, we will have more female role models who will show us that women can be sexy throughout their life span. Until then think of something you like about your body. Then, when you begin to criticize it or feel bad about your appearance, give yourself that positive message.

• *Pessimism.* It is difficult to stay motivated when your expectations of a good outcome are minimal. If sexual dysfunction was an identified problem for you, it will be hard to do some of the exercises when you anticipate only sexual disappointment. Certain sexual problems, like difficulty with orgasm or erection problems, may actually improve as you do some of the exercises. Others, like premature ejaculation or painful intercourse, may require additional efforts. Some good self-help books and a list of organizations that provide referrals to sex therapists can be found listed in the Resources section at the end of this book. Try some of the exercises in this chapter and see if the sexual problems improve. If not, take a break and address the sexual problems before returning to this chapter.

• *Past trauma.* Girls who were sexually abused have had their sexual agency hijacked. It takes a tremendous amount of emotional energy for them to reclaim sexual desire as their own. If you have a history of sexual trauma, it is important that you work through it and understand that what happened to you, although not your fault or your doing, has had an impact on you. It has also had an impact on your sexuality. If you have a history of sexual abuse, taking some time off from having sex can represent an important learning experience. It allows you to start from the beginning in developing and exploring your own sexuality. You may also want to turn to the Resources section for more information on how to move ahead in reclaiming sexual desire.

• *Anger.* If anger with your partner resurfaces during these exercises, it may indicate that the issues that created the anger are not yet fully resolved. Listen to what your desire, or lack of it, is telling you. Step back and do what you need to do to alleviate the stress that is a barrier to your intimate sexual relationship. Entertain the possibility that your anger is being revived as a way to avoid sex and maintain some distance in the relationship. If this is the case, push yourself to do the exercises.

One Step at a Time

You have likely suffered from low sexual desire for quite some time. You may be in a rush to fix it, in order to save the relationship or to save your self-respect. The desire for a quick fix is understandable. But it is not practical. If this problem were easily solved, you would have solved it on your own by now. It is a complex problem and requires time and patience to correct. The way to approach the issue of low desire is to take a gradual approach, one step at a time. Only when you have mastered one step can you proceed to the next. This way you can see where the difficulties lie and where more work needs to be done. If you skip over the exercises, you will be doing yourself a disservice, for it is likely that you will have to go back and repeat and redo things you have already tried. You have probably had enough frustration and "failure," and it will be much more rewarding to feel that you are accomplishing and mastering your desire. If certain exercises do not strike an emotional chord, if they do not directly address your issues with desire, you will master them quickly. But you will still learn something from them. If the exercise is challenging, you will know that it has a great deal of relevance for you, and you can be more confident in the knowledge that the proper groundwork for the next step has been laid.

Most of the time, relationships end when a problem is identified, no solution is offered, and there is no hope of change. Your partner may be unhappy with the lack of sexual intimacy, but he may be gratified by your efforts to deal with it. It means that you take the problem seriously, that you take his feelings seriously, and that there is hope for the future.

9

Sex for Life

Fasten your seat belts. It's going to be a bumpy night.
BETTE DAVIS, *ALL ABOUT EVE*

Once you have reclaimed your sexual interest, you will have changed the sexual balance that was in the relationship. Both you and your partner have sexual interests, desires, and conditions that need to be accommodated. Until this new balance becomes the status quo, it is important to work consciously at maintaining your sexual interest and passion. In this chapter I will present some guidelines for keeping a vital sexual connection with your lover over the long term.

Be True to Your Conditions

Sexual desire is not a given; it needs to be elicited. Remember your conditions for desire, and stick to them. When your conditions for desire are in place, you are more likely to be interested in having sex. Donna's story shows just how important and rewarding it is to be true to your conditions, despite the fact that it often seems easier not to.

154

Donna had a difficult time understanding that she had sexual needs apart from pleasing Michael. She finally came to recognize that she felt desire when she felt good about herself as a competent, capable woman and when she felt close and connected to Michael. On one occasion they had a huge fight about some travel plans Donna had made, and Michael subsequently changed the itinerary behind her back. When Michael initiated sex that evening, Donna was in a quandary. She wanted to put their argument behind them, but she knew that the conditions she had worked so hard to identify were not being met. Donna did not want to have sex. She did not feel close to Michael, and his going behind her back had left her feeling incompetent. So Donna said no to sex, and Michael was upset. In order to stop feeling guilty, Donna kept repeating to herself, "I am not crazy for not wanting sex; I just don't want it right now because I don't feel close or connected to Michael," long after Michael had fallen asleep. The next day, much to Donna's surprise, Michael seemed fine, but *she* still felt guilty. That evening he apologized for changing her airline flight without her consent. Donna felt closer to Michael than she had felt in days. That evening she initiated sex because she really felt desire for her husband. The following day Donna changed her flight plans back to her original plan, chalking up the fees she had to pay to "educational expenses."

Be Assertive

Be clear in word and deed as to when you are sexually interested, when you are not, and when you are open to persuasion. Give up that pattern of avoidance and that reliance on evasive maneuvers.

In order to be assertive, it is important to know what your needs are, to feel entitled to ask for your needs to be met, and to be able to communicate your needs effectively. You are entitled to initiate sex when you feel like it. You are entitled to refuse sex when you don't feel like it. You are also entitled to say maybe or any other response that falls in that gray area between yes and no. Evelyn and Stuart's story demonstrates the value in being assertive about your needs.

Evelyn and Stuart had been married for eighteen years. For much of that time, they had put all their energies into raising the kids and paying the bills. The stress had taken its toll on Evelyn's sexual desire, and Stuart had accepted that this was the way it had to be. But the "kids" were now teenagers, and there was enough money to cover the bills. Evelyn and Stuart now had time for themselves, and their lives were less stressful. Evelyn found it difficult to get interested in sex again, but she didn't want to fight with Stuart, so she would almost always agree to sex when he initiated. But because this was obligatory sex, Evelyn would be easily distracted; she would procrastinate, find excuses to change her mind, or she would simply go through the motions. Stuart got very frustrated. He had no idea when to initiate sex and whether Evelyn was really interested when she responded. He often felt let down and disappointed. He felt inept, unable to figure out how to seduce his wife. Evelyn and Stuart finally came to therapy because they were fighting quite a lot.

Once Evelyn figured out her conditions for desire, she still had to determine in the moment whether she felt like having sex. Then she needed to communicate this to Stuart. One of Evelyn's conditions was that she and Stuart be playful with each other. They decided to incorporate this playfulness into their sexual communication. When Stuart was interested in sex, he would ask Evelyn rather jokingly whether he had a green light. Evelyn felt more comfortable with playful dialogue, and she would respond with either a green light ("Yes"), a red light ("Don't even bother trying"), or a yellow light ("I'm open to persuasion"). The communication was clear and concise, and Stuart and Evelyn ceased fighting about sex.

Treat Your Partner as an Adult

Remember that you are both grown-ups. Your partner is capable of handling difficult feelings and asserting himself so that his needs are met in this relationship.

Yet despite that, women commonly behave as though bolstering her partner's ego for the sake of the relationship is more important than asking for what she needs. In order to have a mutually satisfying sexual relationship, it is often necessary to risk your partner's emotional upset. Men are often extraordinarily uneasy about examining or questioning their sexuality. Women are often uncomfortable seeing their partner struggling, and women often "save" their partner by sacrificing themselves. But grown men are capable of dealing with difficult feelings and changing their behavior as a result. Arlene and Morton's story nicely illustrates the folly of this female sacrifice and the power of changing it.

Arlene left several rather desperate messages for me, asking for help with "menopause-related sexual problems"—specifically, painful intercourse and low sexual desire. When we finally talked on the phone, she told me that she did not think that therapy could help her, but her husband was insistent that she try. Before Arlene stepped into the office, she had already given herself a diagnosis and a prognosis. She was taking the full responsibility for the sexual problems in the relationship, and she was sure that nothing could help her.

This was the second marriage for both Arlene and Morton, and they had been together just ten months. When they met with me, Arlene went out of her way to praise her husband for being so patient with her, so understanding of her problem, and so willing to spend the money for therapy. Morton smiled benignly as his wife sang his praises. He explained to me that he loved Arlene and was willing to be patient with her while she sorted out her problems.

When I met with Arlene alone, a different picture emerged. She confided to me that Morton was a "minute man," very focused on intercourse, with little patience for anything resembling foreplay. Arlene did not want to hurt Morton's feelings, and she did not think she could suggest sexual activities to him for fear of hurting his pride and appearing too sexually demanding. Arlene was willing to sacrifice her sexual pleasure and her sense of herself as a sexual being in order to protect Morton from experiencing himself as a less-than-adequate lover. Morton had no idea that Arlene was unhappy with their lovemaking. He had no idea what Arlene's sexual preferences were, nor did he understand that if he spent more time on "foreplay" activities, she would be more aroused and more lubricated and would enjoy sex more.

In therapy they made changes to their sexual repertoire to include more of the activities Arlene enjoyed. Morton experienced anxiety about his competency as a lover, something he had not thought about for many years. Arlene was uncomfortable seeing her husband struggle to give her pleasure. She put tremendous pressure on herself to experience great passion with the smallest effort Morton expended. It was no wonder she felt little desire. The therapy proceeded more slowly than either Arlene or Morton had originally anticipated. But the slow pace gave them time for their anxieties to subside and allowed for a rebalancing of the relationship with each forward movement. Arlene was finally able to let Morton face his anxieties and conquer them.

And he did. He learned how to be more responsive to Arlene as she became more comfortable telling him what she wanted. About one year after the initial phone call, Arlene and Morton ended treatment, because both were happy with their sexual relationship. Arlene's sexual desire and interest returned, and their lovemaking was less focused on intercourse, to their mutual enjoyment.

Like many women, Arlene bore more than her share of the emotional responsibility in the relationship. She felt that she had to protect Morton from unhappiness, distress, or anxiety, even if it meant taking on the role of the sexually dysfunctional, hormonally unbalanced, troubled partner. Arlene's sacrifice also served her well. After a painful divorce, she wanted a strong man, a man she could depend upon. She did not want to see Morton as being vulnerable or weak or needy in any way. Rebalancing their sexual relationship meant accommodating each partner's anxieties and insecurities about sex, as well as considering each partner's sexual needs, wants, and desires. Change often occurs in "bumpy" steps and often takes more time than we would otherwise anticipate. We need to give ourselves, our partners, and our relationships time to adjust to each step along the way.

Arlene and Morton were lucky. They recognized that there was a problem and sought help quickly. There was little anger between them and their motivation to have a good marriage the second time round sustained them through some anxious moments. Women who have sacrificed their sexuality for extended periods of time often have a lot of anger about this, and the anger is often directed at their partners. Treat your partner as an adult who is capable of handling his feelings and who does not need to be constantly catered to. Continue to focus your efforts and energy on what you can change: you.

Recognize That You and Your Partner May Have Different Views on Sex

There is no absolute right or wrong way to view sex. Find the common ground, and don't get caught up in the game of "who's right?" It is not necessary for your partner to agree that your sexual needs are reasonable, logical, or justified. You must know this. Your partner may feel threatened, insecure, or simply bewildered when you begin to make changes in your life and in your sexual relationship. It is likely that he requires some time to adjust. If you can accept that he may have a different perspective and that your two distinct views can coexist, you will have freed yourself from the need to convince your partner that the changes you are making are right. You do not have to convince your partner that his view of sex is wrong. These types of arguments usually result in couples' feeling more polarized than before. Jennifer and Bill had distinctly different ideas about sex, but once they stopped arguing over who was right, they found a common ground that worked for them.

Jennifer was often tired and stressed at night. She wanted to sleep. Bill thought that the perfect way to relax and unwind at the end of the day was to have sex. Jennifer found this idea absurd and felt that Bill was insensitive just for thinking it. Bill could not understand why Jennifer would not "let herself enjoy sex." He thought her lack of desire was an indication of a deep-seated problem. When Jennifer understood her conditions for having sex (time for herself, with Bill taking care of setting the mood), she did not try to convince Bill that these were important conditions. She simply told him that if he wanted to spend quality time with her, including sex, he would have to take some initiative. This meant doing more of the household tasks and child care so that Jennifer could have some time to herself and so that she would not be too tired to be with Bill. When Jennifer's conditions were met, Jennifer felt strong and assertive, Bill felt loving and generous, and the two spent more intimate (not necessarily always sexual) time together. Bill continued to believe that sex was a great way to relax after a hard day, and Jennifer continued to believe that sleep was the best thing under those conditions.

When You Do Have Sex, Stay Present and Connected

If you have felt that you had no choice but to have sex on your partner's schedule, you may have found yourself being there in body but not in spirit. Certainly your mind may wander during sex, especially if you are preoccupied with something else (a big assignment at work, an upcoming visit from your in-laws, for example). But if you find that you are not mentally present much of the time during sex, take this as a warning sign that something is wrong. Often it means that you are not communicating your needs, your needs are not being met, or you are engaging in obligatory sex. Reclaiming your desire means being able to make a sexual connection with your partner. So if you find that you are just going through the motions, determine what is out of balance, check to make sure that you are being true to your desire conditions, and work on reestablishing a sexual connection. Remember, the desire-arousal feedback loop needs to keep working throughout sex. If you are having trouble staying present during sex, open your eyes and look at your lover, do some focused breathing, and talk to your partner. These are some of the things that helped Cathy.

When Cathy began feeling her own desire again, she was ecstatic. Her sexual relationship with Mark had been fraught with tension for almost three years. Cathy wanted to be sure that she made sex really great, to compensate for lost time and disappointment. She wanted to make sex different and spectacular each time—not because she felt like doing this but because she felt she owed it to Mark. Cathy was falling back into having obligatory sex as a result of the pressure she put herself under. She was becoming disconnected from Mark again. She was not lying back and thinking of England, but she was lying back and thinking of sexually stimulating "tricks." It was not too much longer after this that Cathy again began to lose her interest in sex.

Fortunately, Cathy and Mark were able to see that there was a problem before they were back to square one. Cathy came to understand that she needed to be connected to Mark throughout sex in order to maintain her sexual desire. I told Cathy and Mark to make eye contact and to talk occasionally during lovemaking. I also instructed Cathy to do focused breathing to help her stay present. Ultimately Cathy stopped trying to be a sexual Scheherazade, and she came to experience a deeper sexual connection with Mark.

Deal with the Repercussions of Sexual Trauma

Many women who were sexually abused as children and many women who were assaulted as adults find it difficult to stay present during sex. Often this is because there are certain things that happen during sex, or are associated with sex, that remind them of their abuse. If you were sexually abused and white cotton sheets remind you of the abuse, change them. If a certain sexual position reminds you of the sexual assault, avoid it. Most important, stay present. Although you may be tempted to distract yourself from all that is going on, the connection with your partner will keep you in this moment and out of the past.

If you experience flashbacks of the abuse during sex, please consider seeking the help of a psychologist. A flashback is an intrusive mental picture, emotion, or sensation from the trauma. Although it is a memory, the emotional intensity makes you feel as though you are reliving the traumatic event. Often sex triggers a flashback of sexual abuse or assault. The flashbacks are an indication that the trauma is still very much alive. Some help for your work on sexuality subsequent to assault and abuse can be found in the Resources section at the end of this book. Although I have had a lot of success helping abuse survivors reclaim their sexuality, their happy endings would not have been possible without all the work in therapy that came before.

Natalie had been sexually abused by her father from a very early age until her teen years. Every morning for as long as Natalie could remember, she would go into her parents' bed and cuddle with her father while her mother made breakfast. On many of these occasions, her father would fondle Natalie until she had an orgasm. At first she was not aware that there was anything wrong with this. It felt good. But as she got older, Natalie became increasingly aware that what her father was doing was not right. She began to feel equally complicit and guilty. She told herself, "I should not be doing this. I should not be enjoying this." As time went on, her father was either calling her to his room or seeking her out in hers. They never spoke about what was going on, but Natalie began to feel revolted by her father. Eventually she was able to successfully avoid him. Natalie took comfort in the fact that she seemed able to enjoy sex with her boyfriends, but her negative emotions were revived when she married Sam. She found herself feeling revolted when she was having sex with her husband. The nausea was often overwhelming. Natalie was extremely distressed by this turn of events. She had been in therapy for several years and felt she had really resolved the issues related to the incest. Going step by step over her recent sexual encounters with Sam, we were able to pinpoint the source of Natalie's revulsion. Sam had a rather serious case of five o'clock shadow. When they were dating, Sam always shaved before meeting her. Now that they were married, Sam often had stubble on his face by evening, and the feel of it next to her skin reminded Natalie of her father's face on those mornings when he was abusing her. Sam and Natalie were able to deal with this situation easily, as Sam made a point to shave before he came home from work.

Channel the Sexual Energy You Get Elsewhere Back into the Relationship

When you begin to discover your own sexuality, a whole new world—or an old and long-forgotten world—may open up. Other people may find you sexually appealing, and you may find their interest very exciting, compelling, and tempting. Many of the women I have worked with were tempted at one time or another to have an affair. An affair holds the promise of great excitement. If you are tempted, remember why you started down the road to reclaim your sexuality in the first place. If the motivating force was to improve a troubled relationship, remember that three's a crowd. Mindy came very close to having an affair and ending her relationship with Calvin when she began to focus on her own sexuality instead of on Calvin's premature ejaculation.

> Mindy recognized that one of the consequences of dealing with Calvin's sexual performance was that she had neglected her own sexual desires and preferences. Apart from wanting Calvin to learn better ejaculatory control, Mindy didn't know what her sexual preferences would be, what her conditions for feeling sexual and sexy would be. So she did many of the exercises described in this book. Shortly afterward she requested several individual sessions with me to discuss "a new situation." Mindy had discovered that her boss found her sexually attractive. "I can't believe I didn't see it before," she told me. "Sure, I noticed that he made little jokes here and there, but I never thought anything of it. But now I just know—when he looks at me or talks to me—that he is interested, and I'm afraid that I am, too."
>
> Whether Mindy was correct in assuming that her boss was

interested in having a relationship with her is not the point. She was now feeling more sexual, and she was open to others' perceptions of her as sexual as well. Mindy was truly torn, and she began to flirt with her boss "to test the waters." What initially stopped her from pursuing a relationship with her boss was her anxiety that she would not be good enough in bed, not sexy enough to meet what she thought would be his expectations. Mindy's sexual fantasies about her boss developed as her sexual self-esteem developed. Her awareness of her own sexual attractiveness made her aware of other men's sexuality and other men's appreciation of her. Mindy resisted the temptation to act impulsively and came to realize that although she enjoyed her boss's attention, her desire was not for an affair with him as much as it was a desire to bask in the glow of his admiration.

While it is often tempting to have an affair to shore up one's flagging self-esteem, in the long run, women who have an affair usually end up feeling worse rather than better about themselves. If your partner has found out about the affair, he is bound to feel hurt and betrayed, and you will feel responsible. After an affair it is even more difficult to assert yourself in a positive way and to change things about the relationship that may have prompted the affair in the first place. The balance of power in the relationship ultimately shifts to the "injured" party. Power imbalances can lead to all kinds of relationship problems, including loss of sexual desire, further complicating the picture. Even if the affair goes undiscovered, the deception that is required to cover it up and the guilt one feels about it serve to distance you not only from your partner but also from your true sense of self.

Experiencing yourself as a sexual being can be exciting and uplifting. If you begin to notice that others are attracted to you, or that you are attracted to other people, take this as a positive sign. It means that your sexuality is alive and well. Enjoy the energy you get from your sexuality, and channel that energy back into your relationship. Mindy ultimately used her sexual fantasies about her boss to experience herself as an object of sexual desire and as an agent of sexual passion. Instead of working on a way to have an affair, Mindy brought her newfound sense of sexuality to her relationship with Calvin.

Visualize Changes

Elite athletes often visualize themselves doing something before they actually have to attempt it. It helps them spot potential problems so that they can correct them. It helps them feel confident that they can master the new challenge. This technique can work for sex as well.

When you begin to discover and experience your own sexual desire, interest, and pleasure, you may also experience some anxiety or discomfort. Chances are you are more accustomed to dealing with (or avoiding) your partner's desire but aren't sure what to do with your own. For example, Marissa, who believed that her sexual desire had caused her rape, was more comfortable dealing with Frank's sexual desire and ignoring hers. As long as she was focused on Frank (trying to control where and how he was touching her, while at the same time hoping he was satisfied), she did not have to have or be aware of any sexual desire or interest on her part. As we have discussed elsewhere in the book, many women have been raised to believe that their sexual desire is inappropriate, insignificant, or immoral. It is not surprising that one of the difficulties many women experience is extreme discomfort with their own desire. As Marissa's story illustrates, this is when women can first practice in fantasy what they would like to accomplish in reality. You can use your fantasy sex scene from Chapter 8 to begin, or you can pick up a collection of women's erotic writings to help you along the way.

> When Marissa began experiencing desire and interest in sex, she started to fantasize. What was very distressful to her was the content of her sexual fantasies. She began having very arousing thoughts and images of being coerced, forced, or tricked into having sex. This made Marissa feel that she had indeed wanted to be raped. It was at this point that she experienced one of her frequent urges to stop treatment and revert to having "just get it over with" sex. In therapy Marissa was assured that rape fantasies are one way that women can bypass their own desire in sex. Having fantasies of coercive sex does not mean a woman wants to be raped.
>
> Marissa wanted to get more comfortable with having desire,

so she began reading stories of other women's sexual fantasies. She felt relieved that other women had fantasies of being coerced, but she made a point to masturbate only while reading fantasies that involved women actively desiring sex. She soon found herself becoming aroused to these stories as well. Within a short time, Marissa began having her own sexual fantasies about consensual sex and learning more about what turned her on. She then began to fantasize about what it would be like to be more actively involved in sex with Frank. The more she fantasized about it, the more possible it seemed to her. Marissa eventually felt more comfortable initiating sex and communicating her sexual desires to Frank during sex, since she had already visualized the possibility.

Acknowledge Patterns of Female Sacrifice in Your Family or Friendships

If you find that you are having difficulty making some of the positive changes in your sexual relationship, it can help to look back at the family environment in which you were raised. As women we often feel we must subscribe to culturally prescribed and family-endorsed sexual values such as female selflessness in relationships. This loyalty can make it difficult to capitalize on some of the gains you have achieved in being an equal person, a sexual self, in your relationships. This was certainly the case for Anna.

No woman in Anna's family, as long ago and as far back as her memory could reach, had been happily married. Her mother certainly wasn't, and Anna's own unhappy marriage provided a bond of suffering between the two. Mother and daughter shared an understanding of how difficult men could be. They shared an understanding of how much they had to sacrifice to keep these difficult men. They at least had company in their suffering.

Once Anna became more assertive, and especially once her marriage began to improve, she felt incredibly disloyal. She found that when she was around her mother, she was likely to revert back to complaining about Brian. When she and Brian were around her family together, Anna felt guilty about their intimacy and about Brian's attentiveness to her. It often took several days before Anna could get back to being open in her communication with Brian. He complained of feeling shut out when they were visiting Anna's family, coming back from a visit, or anticipating a visit. Anna felt defensive regarding her family and was frequently tempted to criticize Brian's family "to even things up." The relationship improved again when she told him what she was experiencing. The act of confiding in Brian reinforced the primacy of Anna's bond with him. Anna continued to feel sad about her mother's unhappy marriage, but she ultimately found other ways to connect with her.

As Anna did, the way to avoid this pitfall is to recognize when there is a family pattern of female sacrifice. Often just talking to your mother or aunts or sisters about their relationships can illuminate the pattern. You may need to tolerate the feelings of disloyalty or difference from your family while you work on ways to reinforce a healthier bond with them. You may find that the women in your family also struggled with many of the same issues you face, but they did not feel they had the resources to do anything differently. The best way to acknowledge the selfhood of the women in your family, including yourself, is to respect that they can and did make their own choices about how to manage their relationships. Their choices may not be the same as yours. You do not need to convince them to work on or change or stay within or leave their relationships.

A bond of unhappiness may also be the cement for some of your female friendships. Getting together to complain about the men in your lives may serve to reinforce or justify your sexual disinterest in your partner. Try talking about some of the positive aspects of your partner and your relationship instead, even though it may feel disloyal to your unhappily partnered friends. Respect your friends' choices, but make sure you spend some time talking with and being with happy couples or happily coupled friends.

Stay Tuned In to Your Feelings

We need to pay attention to our feelings, even difficult feelings like anger, anxiety, and loss of sexual desire, all of which give you important feedback about the quality of your life and relationships. If you begin to lose interest in sex again, it is a signal that something in your life is out of balance. Often this imbalance is the same as or similar to the original imbalance you identified in Chapter 3.

Reexperiencing the imbalance does not mean that you have not made progress. On the contrary, you can expect to revisit and address the imbalances in your life on numerous occasions. Each time you will learn a little more and change a little more, until there is a better equilibrium in your life situation.

Michelle had a pattern of avoiding sex by picking an argument or acting grumpy and unattractive in the evenings. Tony had no clue why she seemed so unhappy, and he often tried to make suggestions as to how Michelle could cut down on her workload. This only seemed to make Michelle angrier, and Tony felt hurt that his advice was being rejected. The couple became even more distant from each other. After doing the exercises on her conditions for sex, Michelle recognized that she felt sexy, desirable, and desirous when she felt smart, confident, and independent. So she began to *act* smart, confident, and independent. She took on exciting new challenges at work and told Tony about them. She invited Tony to watch her favorite television show with her, and she began to play music she liked at home. But when Michelle starting initiating sex and paying attention to her own sexual needs and interests during sex, Tony started turning off. The sudden change in the status quo was upsetting to him, and he blamed Michelle, calling her selfish and controlling.

Michelle felt hurt and angry. As for many women, even the suggestion of selfishness was enough to put Michelle on the defensive. She went back to having sex when she thought Tony wanted it, trying to guess when he was in the mood and saying yes when he initiated. She stopped talking about and doing things that were important to her. As it did the first time, this pattern took Michelle further from her own sexual feelings, and her desire plummeted. Since she was reluctant to say no when Tony approached her, she began to avoid Tony again.

When Michelle recognized that she was back where she started, she recommitted to her conditions and to focusing on her own sexual feelings instead of trying to guess at Tony's. In one therapy session Tony told Michelle that it wasn't fair that every time *she* initiated, they had sex, and yet when *he* initiated, it was not a sure thing. "Well," Michelle responded, "what are *your* conditions for sex?" Tony replied that his conditions were that Michelle wanted to have sex with him. "See," she said, "we both have sex when our conditions are met."

Sex Can Be an Important Part of Your Life No Matter What Your Age or Relationship Status

Reclaiming your sexual self involves tapping in to the source of your vitality. Your sexuality is your elixir of life, your own fountain of youth. Not only does your sexuality keep your spirit young, it keeps your relationship vibrant and alive as well. This was a lesson I learned early in my career from a very wise woman.

Barbara was in her early eighties and had been widowed for six months after a sixty-two-year marriage. When she came to my office, I couldn't imagine what she wanted from sex therapy. Perhaps she had been assaulted or traumatized in some way? Maybe she was asking for help for her daughter or granddaughter? But no, this tidy, well-groomed lady, complete with hat and gloves, had come for help with her sexuality. As she explained it to me, she and her husband had had a wonderful sex life. They had been each other's first love and only sexual partner. They had learned about sex together and had enjoyed an active sex life until his death. But far from wanting to bury her sexuality with her husband, Barbara wanted to know how she could keep her sexual vitality. She knew that soon she would want to have a relationship with a man, one that included sex. She knew that emotionally she was not yet ready, nor had she met a man she was interested in, so she wanted to know how she could bridge the gap. Barbara had decided on her own that the answer was masturbation, but she had many questions about it: How did you do it? Was masturbation sufficient to maintain healthy sexual functioning? What exactly was a vibrator, and where could she get one?

I saw Barbara only once, and that was many years ago, but her energy and spirit were impressive. I never knew whether her vitality was a result of her sexuality or whether her sexuality was a result of her vitality. I'm not sure such a chicken-and-egg question is important to answer. It is enough to know that when physical, emotional, and sexual vitality are present, you have all the ingredients for a vibrant, fulfilling life. It is never too late to start. It is always too early to end.

10

Calling on the Professionals

*I know of no more encouraging fact than
the unquestionable ability of man to elevate
his life by a conscious endeavor.*

HENRY DAVID THOREAU, *WALDEN*

All of the couples you have read about in this book came to therapy for help resolving their sexual problems. There was really no other option available to them. Some came for one session, some for several weeks or months, and others worked with me for over a year. While the basic premise of this book is that you can restore sexual passion in your life and in your relationship on your own, there may be good reasons you may also choose to consult a professional.

The Importance of a Physical Exam

For starters, though chances are your trouble isn't physiologically based, it's still important to have a medical checkup. As you read in Chapter 2, there are some physical conditions that can cause or contribute to low sexual desire. Just checking to make sure that you are healthy can eliminate the concern that perhaps your low sex drive is the result of a physical condition that causes general malaise and contributes to low desire. It can save you a lot of time, energy, and stress to first make sure that there is no physical impediment to doing the work described in this book. Think how incredibly demoralizing it would be to try and fail to restore your sexual desire, only to find out later that you had a medical condition that interfered with your progress. This is what happened to Karen.

Karen and Cliff had argued about the low frequency of sex for years. Karen simply did not feel very interested in sex, whereas Cliff felt that he was always interested. Because they loved each other and valued the relationship, they tried many things to revitalize their sexual relationship. They made dates, they read books, they watched movies, and they gave each other massages. Almost everything they tried worked for a while, but soon they would be back to infrequent and, for Karen, obligatory sex.

Karen came to see me on her own, having simply looked in the Yellow Pages for a therapist who treated sexual problems. As part of my normal protocol, I advised her to have a physical examination, something she'd not had for almost five years. It turned out that Karen had a benign growth on her thyroid. Her underactive thyroid had put a stress on her adrenal glands, and Karen was basically "running on empty" almost all the time. Her sexual desire did not magically return when she took thyroid hormone replacement. But she felt less hopeless about the future and less despondent about her past attempts. Karen and Cliff eventually came to therapy together and worked quickly and successfully to restore the passion in their marriage.

Psychotherapy

Perhaps the most compelling reason to consult a psychotherapist is that you are ready to make significant changes in your life and you want some extra help getting started and staying focused. Therapy requires a commitment of time, money, and energy. Dedicating these resources to reclaiming your sexuality is a sign of motivation and provides an additional incentive to make progress.

It is also important to consult a therapist if shame and embarrassment about your situation prevent you from doing the work in this book. An understanding and supportive therapist can help you safely confront issues you may otherwise avoid. Many women make the decision to work on sexual issues when they are in the midst of a crisis. This may mean that the relationship has ended, that the fighting about sex has escalated, or perhaps that the woman or her partner has had an affair. It is also possible that the crisis you are experiencing may have nothing to do with sex but is an additional signal that your life is out of balance. If the crisis, or your life situation, or the fact of having a "sexual problem" makes you feel ashamed or hopeless, it may be helpful at least to talk to a therapist in order to get started.

Sometimes when depression is severe or anxiety is high, these emotions get in the way of your work in this book or, more seriously, interfere with your daily living. It is important to get treatment as soon as symptoms of anxiety or depression appear. Early treatment can reduce the severity and duration of the problem and minimize the chance of recurrences. That said, it is more often the case that people seek treatment *after* a prolonged period of suffering and still achieve significant benefits from therapy. Remember, you need to be in a relatively healthy psychological state before you can begin to effectively do the work in this book. Olivia, whose story is summarized below, was unable to address her low sexual desire until she was in therapy.

Olivia came to see me after Ben left her, telling her that he needed more passion and romance than she had been willing to give him. This was the third significant relationship that Olivia had lost because of her low sexual desire. She was very depressed and felt hopeless about her situation. Before Ben left, Olivia had tried everything she could think of to be more passionate and interested, but nothing she tried seemed to stick. Olivia felt tremendous shame about her three "failed" relationships and hopeless about the prospects of ever marrying. She was having trouble getting out of bed in the morning to go to work, she stopped going to her yoga class, and she declined social invitations from friends. She turned to therapy as a last resort.

Olivia had never really wanted to look at the reasons she lost passion for her lovers once the relationship moved on to a more intimate or committed level. Mostly she expressed the opinion that her lovers should have stuck it out with her, that if they really loved her, they would have been more patient. However, when Ben left, Olivia had to face the fact that the real issue was not her boyfriends' lack of patience but something deeper and even more painful. With the support and guidance she got in therapy, Olivia was able to talk about these issues.

Her mother had left the family to live with another man when Olivia was ten years old, and when that relationship ended, the mother had a series of boyfriends, each more of a "nightmare" than the last, according to Olivia. Years later, when Olivia's father was crippled by a stroke, her mother moved back in to care for him. In therapy Olivia discovered that she was afraid of her passion, fearful that she would end up being like her mother, never having a stable and loving relationship with a good man. She was equally afraid of exploring her anger at her mother, lest she risk her mother's abandonment once again.

It was helpful for Olivia to have a time and a place to explore these painful and, to her, dangerous feelings. Although therapy was a "last resort," it gave her a way of looking at her problems so that she could finally see a way out of her current unhappiness. While dealing with her issues in therapy was difficult for Olivia, it also gave her some much-needed hope. At present Olivia and Ben are corresponding (he had since moved to another state) and discussing the possibility of a future together.

The Right Therapy Works

The best reason to go to therapy is that it actually works. On average, 80 percent of the people who go to therapy end up better off mentally, physically, and emotionally than those who receive no treatment.[1] This is true for people complaining of sexual problems, depression, anxiety, and other mental-health issues. Certain types of therapy work best for certain types of problems. Sex therapy is particularly effective for dealing with sexual problems, because other types of therapy typically consider sexual problems to be merely symptoms of deeper emotional issues. Until the advent of sex therapy, men and women with unhappy sex lives could spend years on the proverbial couch without ever addressing their sexual problems directly. Sex therapy is remarkably effective in helping women achieve orgasm, helping men control the timing of their ejaculation, helping men get and maintain erections, and helping women enjoy pain-free intercourse. And yet neither sex therapy nor other types of therapy have been particularly effective for women or men complaining of low sexual desire. Before exploring how you can use therapy more effectively to improve your sexual desire, it may be helpful to spend a moment considering the factors that have been responsible for reducing its effectiveness.

Why Traditional Therapy Hasn't Worked for Low Sexual Desire

Low sexual desire is not really a sexual dysfunction. Unlike other sexual problems, sexual responses are actually working the way they should in most cases of low desire. Women's sexual desire is extraordinarily sensitive to the emotional environment and to the quality of the relationship. A drop in sexual desire is an early warning signal that something is not right in a woman's life. It is therefore difficult to restore sexual desire by using traditional sex-therapy techniques that assume there is something wrong with the sexual response and that therefore aim to correct it. Treating low sexual desire by prescribing more sex (often in the guise of better sex) usually backfires. It makes women feel worse about themselves and does nothing to address the root problem. At the very best, such limited sex therapy will result in a temporary fix, a "just fake it" approach that rarely if ever improves a woman's life situation. This is what happened to Victoria.

Victoria was a woman in her late forties who had returned to work once her children entered high school. She was excited and interested in her job as an executive secretary. At the same time, her husband, Nigel, was feeling rather jaded about his job in the insurance industry. The children's entering high school seemed to signal to him the approach of the empty nest, and he wanted to concentrate more of his time and energy on the family. Victoria and Nigel went to sex therapy with a colleague of mine because of their increasingly frequent arguments about sex. In therapy Nigel made a compelling case for his view that there was nothing more important to him than his relationships and that he wanted to revive the passion in his marriage. Victoria, perhaps because of her feelings of guilt for wanting a career and "a life outside of my husband and kids," did not give voice to her opinions and so did not make such a positive impression on their therapist. Victoria felt compelled to go along with the agenda of improving their sexual relationship. She and Nigel made dates to do the variety of sexual exercises that the therapist suggested. Nigel habitually asked Victoria, both during and outside of sex, to tell him what he could do to bring her even more sexual pleasure. As Victoria later told me, "I couldn't tell him the truth—that a lot of the time I wanted sex to be quick, that I didn't want it to be a big production all the time. I didn't want to hurt Nigel's feelings, and I knew the therapist wouldn't want to hear that either." Ultimately the sex therapist referred Victoria to me for individual therapy, to deal with her "resistance and fear of intimacy." In individual therapy Victoria was able to talk about how she really felt about sex. Her husband later joined us in therapy (Victoria refused to go back to their joint sex therapist), and we were able to reintegrate sex into their marriage in a way that respected Nigel's wish for connection and Victoria's wish for the connection not to be so all-consuming and, most important, not her responsibility. Victoria and Nigel left therapy with a more flexible relationship than when they started. Sometimes they linger during sex, other times sex is brief and intense, and then again there are times when it is more one-sided, often more focused on Nigel's pleasure but occasionally on Victoria's.

Remember, sex therapists are not experts on what will reignite your passion. You are. A skilled therapist will help you uncover what it is that will work in your unique situation. You need to be honest. If you cannot be honest in front of your partner, request an individual session with the therapist, even if he or she is your "joint" therapist. The goal of this individual time is to work with the therapist to help you share your concerns with your partner in a caring and constructive manner, so that your viewpoint can become part of the therapy. The goal is not to get your therapist to take your side or to keep a secret from your partner. In subsequent therapy sessions your therapist will help you communicate with your partner, letting him in on the discussions in your individual sessions.

While sex therapists may err on the side of advocating more and better sex, sometimes couples counseling takes the other extreme. A technique that is often used (without much lasting success) is asking the higher-desiring partner to abstain from initiating sex until his partner initiates. This strategy is based on the rather outdated notion of sexual desire as simply a drive, which, much like hunger, will be revived after a period of deprivation. What often happens is that a woman's sense of obligation weighs more heavily on her, while her partner's sense of deprivation and frustration grow. This was Samantha's story.

Samantha married her college boyfriend after their graduation and following the discovery of her pregnancy. As Samantha explained, "We were planning on getting married all along, and when I got pregnant, it just didn't seem right to us not to simply move our plans up a few years." Samantha and Neal felt overwhelmed—with a move to a new city, a new apartment, new jobs, a new marriage, and a baby all in one year. They coped as best they could, but their relationship suffered, and Samantha lost her desire for sex.

When their child turned five, Samantha and Neal went to marriage counseling. The counselor advised Neal to stop "pestering" Samantha for sex all the time. She reassured the couple that Samantha's sex drive just needed a rest. For several weeks Samantha and Neal felt happy and optimistic. However, after almost a month, Neal wanted to have sex and felt unhappy that he could not approach Samantha. He wondered how long he was supposed to wait and felt that surely three weeks was more than a reasonable length of time. Samantha knew that she felt no more interested in having sex than she had three weeks earlier. She knew that she "should" initiate sex, but instead she began to avoid Neal so that she could avoid the whole issue of sex. She found new things to complain about regarding Neal and didn't take his unhappiness about sex seriously.

Instead of looking into the problem further, the counselor agreed with Samantha's new complaint that even though Neal wasn't outwardly asking for sex, it was obvious that he wanted to have sex, and his "hangdog look" was continuing to be a turnoff. The message to Neal was that it was not enough to wait for Samantha to initiate sex; he had to erase his own sexual desire from the relationship. Over and again in therapy, the marriage counselor took Samantha's side and admonished Neal to "give his wife more space," to help Samantha around the house, and to express his affection verbally. What happened, tragically, was that Neal found a relationship in which his sexual desire was accepted and acceptable. For years he carried on an affair, finally asking for a divorce when their daughter turned twelve.

Samantha, who is now a psychiatric nurse, believes that the marriage counselor was too much on her side, and she regrets not being pushed to examine her own sexual issues more closely. Samantha came to me for therapy after her divorce to "make sure I don't do the same thing with the next man in my life."

The marriage counselor may have been correct in assuming that Samantha's low desire was due to stress and that she needed time and space to rejuvenate. But the counselor erred in not helping Samantha and Neal find a way to bring sex back into their relationship. Couples therapy and general psychotherapy will often help get at some of the root causes of low desire. Unlike Samantha and Neal, many couples will often feel better about their relationship and will report that their communication and level of intimacy have improved after marital therapy. Despite these improvements, sexual interest and passion are not automatically revived. Similarly, women in individual therapy will often find that their depression lifts, their self-esteem improves, and they are less angry, less anxious, and feel more positive about themselves and their life, but still their sexual passion has not been restored. Why? Talking about sex without examining what your lack of desire means about your life is not effective. Neither is talking about the root causes of your disinterest and avoiding discussions of sex.

Making Therapy More Successful

Given the success of therapy in helping people overcome a myriad of problems, it makes sense to ask what needs to happen to make therapy more helpful to women with low sexual desire. In order to answer this question, it is important to remember that it takes at least two people to make therapy work—the therapist and you (the patient).

The Therapist   There is now some discussion about whether the title "sex therapist" is even an apt moniker for professionals who treat men and women with sexual complaints. I have always referred to myself as a psychologist who specializes in the treatment of sexual problems. I am gratified to see that some other psychologists are doing the same.[2] For those of you who are considering therapy, this is the model I recommend when looking for a therapist—find someone who is an experienced, competent psychotherapist with expertise in treating sexual problems and complaints. This way you can trust that the therapist will understand the reasons for your sexual disinterest and help you translate that understanding into ways of reviving your depressed desire. In other words, you need a skilled therapist who will listen to you and learn from you but who will not, like Samantha's therapist, simply take your side. Your therapist should also help you get a new perspective on your situation and should keep in mind your stated goal of reclaiming your sexual vitality.

Many women with sexual complaints feel more comfortable with a female therapist. They believe that a woman can understand them better, and after all, their complaints are usually related to difficulties with men. The last thing a woman wants is yet another man telling her that she has sexual problems and inadequacies. But this is not what a good therapist of either gender will do. If your therapist has the requisite expertise and knowledge to treat you, she or he will help uncover the source of your low desire and will not pathologize you or pressure you to be sexual with your partner before you are ready. A male therapist may also help you experience a good, safe relationship with a man. Women who have experienced abuse by men in the past or who have issues with control and intimacy related to men are often transformed by a supportive, caring, and safe experience with a male therapist.

Other issues important in determining your choice of therapist will be discussed later in this chapter in the section on finding the right therapist.

You, the Patient   The better prepared you are, the better read you are, and the more you bring to the therapy hour, the more effective your therapy will be. Above all, it is important to listen to your feelings and discuss them with your therapist. If you do not feel comfortable with your therapist and you do not believe it is because he or she is asking you to confront difficult issues, then you may not have a good fit with your current therapist. If you like your therapist but do not think that the type of therapy is working for you, discuss this with your therapist. Many women want interaction with their therapist; they want the therapist to talk to them and to react to them. Typically therapists listen more than they talk, and they do not give advice. While your therapist may give you things to do or think about outside of therapy, he or she will not make important life decisions for you. If you need or want more direction or feedback from your therapist, bring this issue up in therapy. You may be able to resolve the problem. But do not give up on therapy because it doesn't work right the first time. You may have to put some time and energy into choosing the correct therapist and the type of therapy that suits you. I will discuss some of these choices and the factors you should consider later in this chapter.

An important contribution you can make when you go to therapy to get help for your low level of sexual desire is to bring this book with you. Read the book, underline passages that mean something to you (that you agree with, object to, wonder about), and bring in some of your writing exercises to review with your therapist. The exercises in this book are meant to bridge the gap between understanding why your desire is diminished and doing something about it. A good therapist will help you understand what is happening in your life and why. You will be a good patient by being informed about sexual desire problems and by bringing some constructive ideas to the therapy hour. The work you do outside of therapy will make your time with the therapist more productive.

What to Expect from Sex Therapy

When I began doing sex therapy in the early 1980s, I would often encounter worried couples in the hallway outside my office, giggling nervously and anxiously peeking into the office as though they expected to see some large heart-shaped bed in the center of the room. Many men and women expressed concern that they would be required to be sexual in the therapy room. Perhaps lending credibility to this misconception was the fact that in the 1970s and '80s, sexual surrogates were sometimes used by sex therapy clinics to help single patients deal with performance problems. Sexual surrogates could be men but were more often women, who, on the direction of the sex therapist, would participate in completing a set of prescribed sexual exercises with a patient (usually in the patient's home or other private place). The use of sexual surrogates was always controversial, with some critics complaining that surrogates were simply clinically condoned prostitutes. Others argued that surrogates were professionals who could greatly enhance the therapeutic process for very anxious patients with limited opportunities for positive partnered sexual experiences. Nonetheless, sexual surrogates are rarely if ever used today, and many states and professional organizations have deemed their use unethical.

Sex therapy is simply psychotherapy tailored to treat sexual problems and promote healthy sexuality. When you go to sex therapy, you can expect to talk about sex with your therapist, often in some detail. Your therapist needs to understand the ways in which sex works and doesn't work in your relationship. You can also expect to get assignments or exercises to complete at home.

The ease with which the therapist talks about sex may make him or her seem sexually attractive or desirable. Many patients assume that the therapist must have an ideal sex life. Some patients fantasize that their sexual problems would disappear if they had sex with their therapist. You may or may not end up idealizing or fantasizing about your therapist. Do not be upset if you do, but be assured that your therapist cannot be your ideal sexual partner; your therapist cannot be sexual with you at all. It is highly unethical for a therapist to have any sexual contact with his or her patient. An ethical psychotherapist will not touch you in a sexual manner, nor will he or she ever ask you to engage in sex with him or her during or even after the therapy has ended. An ethical therapist will not tell you about his or her sex life. The homework assignments you are given should be consistent with your religious, moral, or personal values. If they are not, you need to consider whether you have adequately conveyed your beliefs to the therapist or whether your therapist does not respect your values. A good therapist will be able to tailor sex therapy assignments so that they reflect and respect the patient's values and beliefs.

In order for therapy to work, you must feel comfortable discussing your sexual thoughts, feelings, and behaviors with your therapist. Dr. Ruth Westheimer made it safe to go into the sex therapy office; talking to Dr. Ruth would be like talking to your grandmother about sex. Although many psychotherapists do not look or act like Dr. Ruth, the fact remains that your therapist, by virtue of his or her demeanor and professionalism, should make you feel safe in the therapy office.

Finding the Right Therapy

What type of professional you decide to consult will determine what type of treatment you receive. The professional help you seek should reflect your understanding of the problem and your personal preferences. For example, after doing the work in the first couple of chapters of this book, you may be convinced that the source of your problem is an imbalance of power in your relationship. If you want to consult a professional in addition to doing the work in this book, you may want to look for a therapist you and your partner could see together. On the other hand, if you think that the root problem is difficulties with intimacy, you may feel more comfortable going to see a therapist alone, at least for a while. Or your preference still may be to work on intimacy issues with your partner and go to therapy together.

This decision will be based on your preference and your comfort level. Here are some general guidelines to consider:

- Consider going into therapy with your partner if you believe that your low desire is related to an imbalance in control and power, stress, or unresolved anger.

- Consider at least starting therapy on your own if the issues are related to intimacy or sexual self-esteem.

- If you or your partner has a sexual problem that has caused you to lose desire, then absolutely see a therapist who has skill and expertise in treating sexual problems. This therapist will want to see you as a couple, at least for an evaluation of the problem.

- If you believe that your low desire is a result, even in part, of unresolved trauma in your background, you will be best served by seeing a therapist who is skilled in dealing with trauma. It is preferable to deal with these issues individually before trying to deal with them as a couple.

- If you believe that you are in a bad relationship, if you are considering leaving the relationship, but especially if you are concerned that it is an abusive relationship, you should seek therapy on your own. Do not include your partner.

- If you are convinced that your low desire has some physical origin, you will certainly want to consult a physician. Your gynecologist is probably the first physician to talk to.

- If you have other emotional issues that are interfering with your life, your sexuality, and your work in this book, please consult a psychologist and discuss the possibility of a referral to a psychiatrist for an evaluation of whether medication would be helpful.

The Right Therapist for You

You may be fortunate enough to have a physician or a gynecologist whom you feel comfortable asking for a referral. Another source of referral information can be state (or, in Canada, provincial) psychological associations, as well as other mental health associations.

Many of these groups have a list of licensed psychotherapists grouped by specialty and geographic area. Contact information can be found in Appendix B. While it is best to get a referral from someone you trust (either a person or an agency), sometimes the Yellow Pages are the best you can do. Regardless of the source of the name of a prospective therapist, it is ultimately up to you to choose.

There are many different disciplines that train therapists: psychiatry, psychology, social work, and counseling. Psychiatrists are medical doctors who have done advanced training (residency) in treating mental illness. Because they are physicians, psychiatrists can prescribe medications. If you are considering antidepressants or antianxiety medication, it is important to consult a psychiatrist and not rely on your general practitioner to write you a prescription. A psychiatrist has expertise in prescribing medication that will most effectively target the symptoms you are experiencing. Many psychiatrists conduct therapy in addition to prescribing medication, and their medical background lends itself well to the treatment of mental or emotional disorders that are biologically based, such as severe depression, schizophrenia, and bipolar disorder.

Psychologists typically have a doctoral-level degree (a Ph.D., Psy.D., or Ed.D.) in clinical or counseling psychology. In essence they have at minimum four or more years of postgraduate study. Psychologists follow a scientist-practitioner model, and generally their treatment is informed by their knowledge and understanding of clinical research. Clinical social workers and counselors generally have about two years of postgraduate education and hold master's degrees. In addition to meeting educational requirements, psychologists, social workers, and counselors have to have some period of supervised practice before they are licensed to practice independently.

When choosing a therapist, you should consider the person's education level (master's or doctorate), field of study (psychology, social work, or counseling), and unless you are going to a hospital- or clinic-based therapist, you should insist on a licensed professional. The fees that psychotherapists charge are generally in line with their education and training. Psychiatrists usually charge the most, followed by psychologists, social workers, and counselors, in that order. Traditional insurance plans that cover psychotherapy almost always cover the services of psychiatrists and licensed psychologists (at least in part). Many now cover the services of social workers and other licensed professionals, but check with your insurance carrier first.

Treating sexual problems requires an understanding of the complex interplay between psychology, physiology, and intimate relationships. You want to be certain that the professional you choose to see has experience, expertise, education, and training specifically regarding the treatment of sexual problems. There is no licensure for "sex therapists." While some organizations may provide a certification, this simply means that the individual has satisfied that organization's criteria, which may range from simply joining the organization to meeting some educational or experiential standards. You can also find out whether a therapist has the expertise to help you by asking him or her these simple questions when you make that first phone call:

- Do you have experience treating people with sexual problems?
- Have you treated people with low sexual desire?
- What is your general approach to treating low sexual desire?
- Can you tell me something about your educational background or your training in the field of sex therapy?

How the therapist responds to these questions will help you determine whether he or she is capable and experienced and whether you will feel comfortable at least setting up an initial appointment. Be wary of therapists who guarantee success, who tell you how long therapy will last, or who are offended by the questions. You are the consumer, and you have a right to ask.

If you felt positive about the therapist's responses to your questions during the initial phone call, take the next step and ask for a consultation or an appointment. You are not committed to anything. While most therapists will charge you for this appointment, you are not signing on the dotted line for anything other than a simple visit. Make sure before scheduling the appointment that the therapist is accepting new patients for ongoing therapy. It is very disheartening to have that first consultation and really connect with a therapist, only to discover that he or she could see you only for that one visit. While much of that initial visit will involve telling the therapist about yourself, take some time to ask the therapist more questions. Relevant questions include these:

- How do you work in therapy? It is important to me to know what you are thinking or how you view my situation. Is that something you do in therapy?
- Do you ever recommend books? Do you give assignments in therapy?
- How often would you want to see me?
- How long does therapy typically last?
- What is your policy about cancellations, missed appointments, and vacations?
- Do you work with a psychiatrist or other medical doctor who prescribes medication?
- What is your feeling about medication for sexual desire problems?

Therapy Doesn't Have to Be Forever

The specific focus of sex therapy typically makes the overall duration of therapy shorter than therapy that is directed at chronic depression or anxiety. Treatment for sexual problems usually lasts less than a year. How long therapy takes for you and/or your partner will depend on the nature and the severity of the issues that underlie your low desire. You may also choose to set up consultation appointments rather than ongoing therapy. When you ask for a consultation, the understanding is that you want to have several visits with a psychotherapist to discuss a particular issue. For example, you may want to consult a therapist to help you reflect upon your answers to the questionnaire in Chapter 3 and to have a professional opinion weigh in on what the imbalance is in your life. Or you may feel that you are stuck at a certain point when you are doing the exercises and want some help understanding the problem and moving ahead. I often do consultations for people who are in general psychotherapy with someone else and who want to talk to an expert about their sexual issues. Once we have discussed their sexual concerns, they take what they have gained from the consultation back into their therapy. So if you are already in therapy, you do not need to change therapists to deal with your low desire. You can bring your work from this book with you to your therapist and, if needed, get a consultation with a sex expert to help your therapy progress.

Many people find therapy so helpful that they choose to maintain a relationship with their therapist even after the sexual problems are resolved. They may not come for weekly sessions, but they find it helpful and reassuring to have a professional to turn to when they are encountering difficulties in their lives. I have several clients with whom I have an ongoing relationship of over fifteen years. Years may go by when I do not see them or hear from them, but then they call when they are encountering some new life challenge.

Therapy for Trauma

Women who have suffered trauma (sexual or otherwise) often need to resolve the trauma in individual therapy before working on their sexual desire. In the past this may have meant years in therapy. Now psychotherapy can offer new approaches to trauma that dramatically reduce the time spent in therapy and the pain involved in recalling and working on traumatic memories. The most researched and relevant of these techniques is called Eye Movement Desensitization and Reprocessing, or EMDR.

EMDR is based on the premise that our central nervous system has a built-in mechanism for processing life events that promotes our psychological development and helps us deal with the small traumas that are an inevitable part of living. However, our capacity to adapt and grow is sometimes overwhelmed by serious trauma or by lesser traumatic events if they occur at a particularly vulnerable point in our lives (especially childhood). Therapists who use EMDR ask the patient to call up the traumatic memory in all its manifestations: visual, cognitive, emotional, and physical. The therapist then guides the patient to move his or her eyes back and forth in a manner that mimics the eye movements that occur in REM sleep. The theory is that the eye movements stimulate our natural adaptive system to accelerate recovery and healing.

Research supports the effectiveness of EMDR, with studies showing complete symptom remission in as little as three sessions of EMDR in patients with a history of trauma.[3] My own clinical experience supports this, as Mary's case illustrates.

Mary is a woman in her mid-thirties who came to see me complaining of recurrent vaginal infections and painful intercourse that was not helped by medical treatments. Mary avoided sex and had essentially lost her desire for sex because of the pain she experienced. A male teacher had raped Mary when she was in the second grade, and she wondered whether the trauma could be relevant to her sexual problems. Mary had never been in therapy before, but she had felt that she had resolved the issue of her abuse by attending AA meetings for her alcoholism. Recently she was experiencing great anxiety and discomfort, since her daughter had entered the second grade. While her daughter had a perfectly lovely female teacher, Mary was concerned about her daughter's male phys-ed teacher, her male gymnastics coach, and indeed all adult males outside the family. Mary began to experience flashbacks—recurrent, distressing images of her rape that would leave her shaking and sobbing.

In the first session of EMDR, Mary recalled the terror and the powerlessness she felt during the rape. Soon her shaking and sobbing was replaced by a fierce anger: "How could he do that to me? I want to kill him." She left the session feeling that although she was powerless as a child to prevent or stop the assault, she was not powerless as an adult. She felt confident that she could protect her daughter in a way that she herself had not been protected. Mary reported that she felt calm all week.

In her next EMDR session, Mary focused on the pain in her vagina. She immediately began to get images of the rape and started to cry and shake. She reported feeling that she was being ripped apart and feeling as if she would die. Mary continued to cry and feel that she was damaged. By the end of the session, however, she reported seeing images of her daughter being born, and she started to think about the damage as having occurred in the past. She took great pride in the fact that her body had worked well to produce a healthy baby girl. Mary left the session smiling.

The next few sessions of EMDR continued to focus on Mary's feelings of power, health, and healing. In one session, she reported the feeling that her vagina was small, too small for a penis to enter. Quickly, however, she recalled the birth of her daughter and the times early in her relationship with her husband when intercourse had not been painful, and she began to visualize her vagina as a healthy part of her body and to see herself as able to engage in pleasurable sexual intercourse if she wanted to.

After six sessions of EMDR, Mary was able to address her pain by utilizing the sex therapy techniques she had previously resisted. She and her husband were able to regularly have pain-free intercourse within three months of Mary's initial appointment. Mary continued to work on other issues in therapy. She was very hard on herself at the office, rather controlling in her intimate relationships, and overprotective as a mother. But Mary's whole outlook had changed. She approached therapy very positively and knew that she could and would make positive changes in her life.

EMDR is best used as part of a comprehensive treatment approach and in the context of a good therapeutic relationship. For people with a history of trauma, it can be invaluable in helping them move forward in therapy more quickly than they otherwise might.

Beyond Problems and on to Enhancing Your Physical and Mental Health

In addition to its success helping people overcome a variety of problems, psychotherapy can also be used to promote a sense of personal well-being and happiness. Many people use their weekly or biweekly sessions with a therapist to examine their life and make conscious choices. When people feel in charge of their lives and feel they have made good decisions for themselves, they become happier and more satisfied. As I've said before, the better you feel about yourself and your life, the more likely it is that you will feel sexual desire. There are many options available to you if peak physical and mental health is a priority.

While your doctor can certainly help you rule out physical problems, you can also turn to alternative therapies to help you maximize your health and get your body working at an optimal level. If you want good nutritional advice, see a nutritionist. He or she can evaluate your diet, make food recommendations, and suggest vitamins and nutritional supplements that can improve your general sense of physical well-being. Other women find massage therapy, acupuncture, yoga, or meditation helpful. Alternative or holistic therapies work to build up the body's own healing process. Being in good physical, mental, and emotional shape will go a long way to helping you restore your sexual desires.

Beware of the Medicalization of Sex and Sex Therapy

Being an informed consumer is the best way to find a qualified professional to help you restore your sexual desire. In your quest you will no doubt come across advertisements, prescriptions, and promotions for creams, pills, patches, and pumps to help you boost your flagging desire. Just look at the huge industry for diet aids and supplements (most of which are not effective in the long run and some of which are downright dangerous) to see where the sexual desire market is heading.

Drug companies are currently spending millions of dollars on marketing campaigns aimed at getting physicians to buy into the notion that women's sexual problems are likely to have a physical basis. If they are successful, physicians will be a potentially lucrative market for the medications the industry hopes to soon have available. In the meantime do not get drawn into having expensive diagnostic tests performed at one of the several sexual medicine centers that have recently arisen. Your physician should have a strong rationale for sending you for expensive tests that risk increasing your anxiety and sense of alienation from your body and your sexuality. Your physician may prescribe a drug or order a test because he or she genuinely wants to help and feels that this is all there is to offer. It is a sad reality that the most training many doctors have had regarding human sexuality is that provided by a drug-company representative or spokesperson. Your physician should also be able to provide you with recommendations for qualified professionals to talk to regarding your concerns about sexual desire. If he or she does, you can have more confidence that your doctor has a balanced understanding of the complexities of sexual desire.

Calling on the Professionals: A Checklist

☐ Even if you don't believe that your problems are physiological, get a physical exam to ensure that there are no medical problems that would interfere with your progress.

☐ Get a referral from your doctor or an agency, or look in the Yellow Pages to get the names of experienced psychotherapists who deal with sexual problems. Ideally, get several names.

☐ Interview prospective therapists on the telephone.

☐ Make an appointment for an initial visit with one or two therapists you felt the most comfortable with on the telephone.

☐ Choose a therapist based on your evaluation of his or her ability to help you and the comfort you felt in the session.

☐ Bring this book with you to therapy. The more work you do, the more effective your therapy will be.

☐ Consider adjunctive therapies such as nutrition, massage, exercise, or movement therapy in order to maximize your well-being.

Maintain a healthy optimism. You can reclaim your sexual self!

Notes

Introduction

1. Michael, Robert T., John H. Gagnon, Edward O. Laumann, and Gina Kolata. *Sex in America: A Definitive Survey* (New York: Warner Books, 1995).
2. Masters, William H., and Virginia E. Johnson. *Human Sexual Response.* (Boston: Little, Brown, 1966).
3. Northrup, Christiane. *The Wisdom of Menopause* (New York: Bantam Books, 2001).
4. Michael, Robert T., et al. *Sex in America.*

1: Sex Doesn't Exist in a Vacuum

1. Laumann, Edward O., John H. Gagnon, and Robert T. Michael. *Sex, Love and Health in America* (Chicago: University of Chicago Press, 2001).
2. The results of the National Health and Social Life survey data set are reported in Laumann, *Sex, Love and Health in America.*
3. Tolman, Deborah. "Female Adolescent Sexuality: An Argument for a Developmental Perspective on the New View of Women's Sexual Problems." In Ellyn Kaschak and Leonore Tiefer (eds.), *A New View of Women's Sexual Problems* (New York: Haworth Press, 2001).
4. These surveys are reported in Regan, P. C., and E. Berscheid, *Lust: What We Know About Human Sexual Desire* (Thousand Oaks, Calif.: Sage, 1999).
5. Ibid., p. 79.
6. This term was first used to describe sexual scripts by Judith Daniluk in *Women's Sexuality Across the Lifespan* (New York: Guilford, 1998).

2: Could the Trouble Be Physical?

1. Daniluk. *Women's Sexuality Across the Lifespan.*
2. Kingsberg, S. A. "The Impact of Aging on Sexual Function in Women and Their Partners." *Archives of Sexual Behavior* 31 (2002): 431–437.
3. Northrup. *The Wisdom of Menopause.*
4. Ibid.
5. The National Council on Aging. *Healthy Sexuality and Vital Aging* (September 1998).

6. Reichman, Judith. *I'm Not in the Mood: What Every Woman Should Know About Improving Her Libido* (New York: Quill, 1998).

7. Reinisch, June. *The Kinsey Institute New Report on Sex* (New York: St. Martin's Press, 1990).

8. Berman, Jennifer, and Laura Berman. *For Women Only: A Revolutionary Guide to Overcoming Sexual Dysfunction and Reclaiming Your Sex Life* (New York: Henry Holt, 2001).

9. Sherwin, B. S. "Randomized Clinical Trials of Combined Estrogen-Androgen Preparations: Effects on Sexual Functioning." *Fertility and Sterility* 77, no. 2 (2002): 49–54.

3: Why Don't I Feel the Way I Used to Feel?

1. Hochschild, Arlie R. *The Second Shift: Working Parents and the Revolution at Home.* (New York: Viking Press, 1989).

2. Fogarty, T. "On Emptiness and Closeness." In Eileen G. Pendegast (ed.), *The Family.* (New Rochelle, N.Y.: Center for Family Learning, 1979).

3. Ellison, Carol Rinkleib. *Women's Sexualities* (Oakland, Calif.: New Harbinger Publications, 2000).

4. Reissman, Catherine Kohler. *Divorce Talk: Women and Men Make Sense of Personal Relationships* (New Brunswick, N.J.: Rutgers University Press, 1990).

5. Berliner, L., and D. M. Elliott. "Sexual Abuse of Children." In John Myers, Lucy Berliner, John Briere, Carole Jenny, C. Terry Hendrix, and Theresa Reid (eds.), *The APSAC Handbook on Child Maltreatment,* 2nd ed. (Thousand Oaks, Calif.: Sage, 2001).

6. Adapted from a handout produced by Womanspace, Trenton, N.J.

4: Taking Stock: What Are You Saying When You Are Saying No?

1. Kent, Jack. *There's No Such Thing as a Dragon* (New York: Golden Press, 1975).

5: Reclaiming Your Sexual Self

1. Barbach, Lonnie. *For Yourself: The Fulfillment of Female Sexuality* (New York: Doubleday, 1975).

2. Zilbergeld, Bernie. "Some Nonstandard Deviations from the Current Thinking in the Sex Profession." Panel presented at the annual meeting of the Association of Sex Educators, Counselors, and Therapists, Las Vegas, 1981.

6: When Is Sex Right for You?

1. Lerner, H. *The Dance of Anger: A Woman's Guide to Changing the Patterns of Intimate Relationships* (New York: HarperCollins, 1997).

7: Getting Your Signals Straight: It's All about Communication

1. Levine, Judith. *Harmful to Minors: The Perils of Protecting Children from Sex* (Minneapolis: University of Minnesota Press, 2002).

2. Ibid., p. 135.

3. Tannen, Deborah. *You Just Don't Understand: Women and Men in Conversation* (New York: Ballantine, 1990).

8: Sexercises for the Mind and Body

1. Krucoff, Carol, and Mitchell Krucoff. *Healing Moves: How to Cure, Relieve, and Prevent Common Ailments with Exercise* (New York: Harmony Books, 2000).
2. Nelson, Miriam. *Strong Women Stay Young.* (New York: Bantam, 1988).

10: Calling on the Professionals

1. Donahey, K. M., and S. D. Miller. "What Works in Sex Therapy: A Common Factors Perspective." In Kleinplatz, Peggy J. (ed.), *New Directions in Sex Therapy: Innovations and Alternatives* (Philadelphia, Pa.: Brunner-Routledge, 2001).
2. Ellison, Carol Rinkleib. "Intimacy-Based Sex Therapy: Sexual Choreography." In *Women's Sexualities* (Oakland, Calif.: New Harbinger Publications, 2000).
3. Wilson, S. L. A., and R. H. Becker. "Eye Movement Desensitization and Reprocessing (EMDR) Treatment for Psychologically Traumatized Individuals." *Journal of Consulting and Clinical Psychology* 63 (1995): 928–937; and Wilson, S. A., L. A. Becker, and R. H. Tinker. "Fifteen Month Follow-up of Eye Movement Desensitization and Reprocessing (EMDR) Treatment for Posttraumatic Stress Disorder and Psychological Trauma." *Journal of Consulting and Clinical Psychology* 65 (1997): 1047–1056.

Appendix A:
Sex Hormones

Estrogens

Estrogens comprise the group of hormones known as the female hormones because of their importance in stimulating the development of the reproductive structures and secondary sex characteristics in women. The hormone of greatest interest is estradiol, which is manufactured mainly by the ovaries in women and by the testes in men. Women have much higher amounts of estrogen than do men. The estrogens are important in terms of sexual functioning because they maintain vaginal elasticity and prevent and relieve vaginal dryness in women, but they do not appear to directly affect sexual desire in either men or women.

Progesterone

This hormone is seen in higher levels in women than in men. Progesterone levels fluctuate during the menstrual cycle but peak after ovulation and remain high until a few days before menstruation. Progesterone is responsible for preparing the endometrial lining of the uterus to receive a fertilized egg. The progesterone levels of sexually interested and disinterested women have not been found to differ, but there is evidence that giving progesterone to either men or women decreases sexual desire.

Prolactin

Prolactin is produced by the pituitary gland and is important in promoting growth in both men and women. It also promotes the development of breast tissue, stimulates the production of milk for new mothers, and inhibits ovulation (but does not necessarily prevent it, making breast-feeding an unreliable contraceptive option). What role prolactin plays in sexual desire is unclear. Researchers have found that men and women with abnormally high levels of prolactin have low levels of sexual desire. However, the reverse is not necessarily true, and women with low sexual desire most often have normal levels of this hormone.

Androgens

This group of hormones is known as the male hormones. Androgen levels are higher in men than in women, and the androgens are responsible for the development of the male secondary sex characteristics. Testosterone, androstendedione, and dehydroepiandrosterone (DHEA) are included in this group. Testosterone is the most widely known and researched of the androgens, and the data about its effects are mixed. We do not as yet know what the normal range of testosterone levels is in women, as this has not been well studied or documented. What is known is that some amount of this hormone is necessary for sexual desire to be experienced. Women who experience a reduction in testosterone (usually related to having their ovaries removed) often also experience a reduction in their desire for sex, which is restored with testosterone therapy.

Sex Hormone Binding Globulin (SHBG)

It is the amount of each hormone that is available for our bodies' use that is important. Available levels of testosterone and estrogen are interdependent. Estrogen stimulates our bodies' production of a protein called sex hormone binding globulin or SHBG. SHBG binds to both estrogen and testosterone, thereby restricting the availability of both hormones. Since SHBG binds more readily to testosterone, increasing levels of estrogen will result in decreased levels of available or "free" testosterone.* Likewise, increased levels of testosterone are countered by the body's production of more estrogen. There are many sources of both estrogen and testosterone in the female body. It is noteworthy that the brain converts a portion of testosterone to estradiol. It appears that our bodies strive for some optimal balance between these two vital hormones.

* Reichman, J. *I'm Not in the Mood: What Every Woman Should Know about Improving Her Libido* (New York: Quill, 1998).

Appendix B: Medications That Can Decrease Sexual Desire

Please note that this list is intended to be as comprehensive as possible.* You may or may not experience any noted side effect of a medication. Some of these medications may decrease desire because of adverse effects on mood or sexual performance. Also, the fact that a medication you are using is *not* listed here does not mean that your low desire is not related to your use of it. I have not included all of the numerous medications that list loss of desire as a rare side effect. If you suspect that your loss of desire is due to or related at least in part to the medication you are taking, consult your physician. Do not discontinue a medication without consulting your doctor.

Class	Generic Name	Brand Name	Uses
Antihypertensives	Clonidine hydrochloride	Catapres Dixarit (in Canada)	To relieve high blood pressure
	Clonidine hydrochloride and Chlorthalidone	Clorpres	To relieve high blood pressure; diuretic

(continued on next page)

* This list was compiled from various resources including: *2004 Physicians' Desk Reference* (Montvale, N.J.: Thomson PDR, 2003); Sifton, D. (ed.). *PDR Drug Guide for Mental Health Professionals* (Montvale, N.J.: Thomson Medical Economics, 2002); Foley, S., S. A. Kope, and D. P. Sugrue. *Sex Matters for Women* (New York: Guilford Press, 2002); Leiblum, S. R., and R. C. Rosen (eds.). *Sexual Desire Disorders* (New York, Guilford Press, 1988); and MEDLINE Plus Health Information, an Internet service of the U.S. National Library of Medicine and the National Institutes of Health at www.nlm.nih.gov/medlineplus/druginfo, last accessed on January 5, 2004.

Class	Generic Name	Brand Name	Uses
	Chlorthalidone	Hygroton Thalitone Apo-Chlorthalidome (in Canada) Novo-Thalidone (in Canada) Uridon (in Canada)	Diuretic; to relieve high blood pressure
	Guanethidine	Ismelin Apo-Guanethidine (in Canada)	To relieve high blood pressure
	Hydrochloro-thiazide	Esidrix Hydro-chlor Hydro-D HydroDiuril Microzide Oretic Apo-Hydro (in Canada) Diuchlor H (in Canada) Neo-Codema (in Canada) Novo-Hydrazide (in Canada) Urozide (in Canada)	Diuretic; to relieve high blood pressure
	Lisinopril	Prinivil Zestril	To relieve high blood pressure; vasodilator to treat congestive heart failure
	Methyldopa	Aldomet Apo-Methyldopa (in Canada) Dopamet (in Canada) Novomedopa (in Canada) Nu-Medopa (in Canada)	To relieve high blood pressure
	Methyldopa and Chlorothiazide	Aldochlor Supres (in Canada)	To relieve high blood pressure
	Methyldopa and Hydrochloro-thiazide	Aldoril Novodoparil (in Canada) PMS Dopazide (in Canada)	To relieve high blood pressure

Class	Generic Name	Brand Name	Uses
	Metoprolol	Lopressor Toprol-XL Apo-Metoprolol (in Canada) Betaloc (in Canada) Novometoprol (in Canada) Nu-Metop (in Canada)	To relieve high blood pressure; to treat various cardiac conditions
	Prazosin	Minipress	To relieve high blood pressure; to treat congestive heart failure and Raynaud's disease
	Propranolol	Inderal Inderal LA Apo-Propranolol (in Canada) Detensol (in Canada) Novopranol (in Canada) pms-Propranolol (in Canada)	To relieve high blood pressure
	Reserpine	Serpalan Novoreserpine (in Canada) Reserfia (in Canada) Serpasil (in Canada)	To relieve high blood pressure; off-label uses include treatment of Raynaud's disease. (Side effects with reserpine may occur after you stop using the medication)
	Spironolactone	Aldactone Novospiroton (in Canada)	Diuretic; to relieve high blood pressure; off-label uses include treatment of polycystic ovary syndrome and hirsutism
	Spironalactone and Hydro-chlorothiazide	Aldactazide Novo-Spirozine (in Canada)	Diuretic; to relieve high blood pressure

(continued on next page)

Class	Generic Name	Brand Name	Uses
Heart Medication	Digoxin	Lanoxin Lanoxicaps Novo-Digoxin (in Canada)	To improve the strength and efficiency of the heart and to control heartbeat rate and rhythm
Antidepressants/ MAO Inhibitors	Phenelzine	Nardil	To treat depression
Tricyclics	Amitriptyline	Elavil Endep Levate (in Canada) Novotriptyn (in Canada)	To treat depression
	Amoxapine	Asendin	To treat depression
	Clomipramine	Anafranil	To treat depression; off-label uses include treatment of bulimia, narcolepsy, neurogenic pain disorder, and panic disorder
	Imipramine	Norfranil Tipramine Tofranil Apo-Imipramine (in Canada) Novopramine (in Canada)	To treat depression
	Protriptylene	Vivactil Triptil (in Canada)	To treat depression, narcolepsy, and cataplexy
	Citalopram	Celexa	To treat depression
SSRIs	Fluoxetine	Prozac Sarafem	To treat depression and premenstrual dysphoric disorder (more commonly referred to as PMS)
	Paroxetene	Paxil Paxil CR	To treat depression, obsessive-compulsive disorder, anxiety disorders, and post-traumatic stress disorder

Class	Generic Name	Brand Name	Uses
	Sertraline	Zoloft	To treat depression, obsessive-compulsive disorder, anxiety disorders, and post-traumatic stress disorder
Other Antidepressants	Bupropion	Wellbutrin Zyban	To treat depression and to help stop smoking (increased sexual desire is also a noted side effect)
	Venlafaxine	Effexor Effexor XR	To treat depression
Antimanic	Lithium	Cibalith-S Eskalith Lithane Lithobid Lithonate Lithotabs Carbolith (in Canada) Duralith (in Canada) Lithizine (in Canada)	To treat mania, especially the manic phase of bipolar disorder
Neuroleptics	Chlorpromazine	Thorazine Largactil (in Canada) Novochlorpromazine (in Canada)	Antipsychotic
	Haloperidol	Haldol Apo-Haloperidol (in Canada) Novo-Peridol (in Canada) Peridol (in Canada) PMS Haloperidol (in Canada)	Antipsychotic, for control of muscular tics associated with Tourette's syndrome, and for the treatment of symptoms related to Huntington's chorea
	Thioridazine	Mellaril Apo-Thioridizine (in Canada) Novo-Ridazine (in Canada) PMS Thioridazine (in Canada)	To treat schizophrenia and symptoms related to Huntington's chorea; also acts as a sedative

(continued on next page)

Class	Generic Name	Brand Name	Uses
	Thiothixene	Navane	Antipsychotic
	Fluphenazine	Permitil	Antipsychotic and
		Proloxin	antineuralgic
		Apo-Fluphenazine (in Canada)	adjunct
		Modecate (in Canada)	
		Moditen (in Canada)	
	Risperidone	Risperdal	Antipsychotic
	Prochlorperazine	Compazine	Antipsychotic and
		Nu-Prochlor (in Canada)	antiemetic agent
		PMS Prochlorperazine (in Canada)	
		Stemetil (in Canada)	
Minor Tranquilizers	Alprazolam	Alprazolam-Intensol Xanax	To relieve anxiety
		Alti-Alprazolam (in Canada)	
		Apo-Alpraz (in Canada)	
		Gen-Alprazolam (in Canada)	
		Novo-Alprazol (in Canada)	
		Nu-Alpraz (in Canada)	
	Diazepam	Valium	To relieve anxiety,
		Apo-Diazepam (in Canada)	muscle spasms,
		Diazemuls (in Canada)	and seizures
		Novo-Dipam (in Canada)	
		PMS-Diazepam (in Canada)	
		Vivol (in Canada)	
	Clorazepate	Tranxene	To relieve anxiety,
		Apo-Clorazepate (in Canada)	muscle spasms,
		Novo-Clopate (in Canada)	and seizures

Class	Generic Name	Brand Name	Uses
	Lorazepam	Ativan Lorazepam Intensol Apo-Lorazepam (in Canada) Novo-Lorazem (in Canada) Nu-Loraz (in Canada)	Uses include: antianxiety, antiemetic, anticonvulsant, muscle relaxant, antitremor, and sedative
	Phenobarbital	Luminol Solfoton Ancalixir (in Canada)	To relieve anxiety; short-term treatment of insomnia
Hormones	Bicalutamide	Casodex	To treat prostate cancer
	Crinone	Crinone Gesterol 50 Prometrium PMS-Progesterone (in Canada)	To regulate menstrual cycle To help or maintain a pregnancy; added to estrogen replacement to prevent thickening of the uterus; to treat endometriosis; to treat breast, kidney, and uterine cancer; to treat appetite loss due to AIDS
	Finasteride	Propecia Proscar	Used in treatment of benign enlargement of prostate; to promote hair growth in men
	Flutamide	Eulexin	Antiandrogen used to treat prostate cancer
	Goserelin	Zoladex	To treat prostate cancer, endometriosis, advanced breast cancer in premenopausal women
	Interferon Alfacon-1	Infergen	Prevents growth of hepatitis C virus

(continued on next page)

Class	Name	Brand Names	Uses
	Leuprolide	Lupron Lupron Depot Viadur	To treat uterine bleeding; for pain due to endometriosis; to treat infertility and prostate cancer
	Nafarelin	Synarel	To treat symptoms of endometriosis— e.g., pelvic pain, muscle cramps, and painful intercourse
	Nilutamide	Nilandron Anandron (in Canada)	Antiandrogen, used to treat prostate cancer (with surgical removal of testicles)
	Nolvadex	Tamoxifen Apo-Tamox (in Canada) Gen-Tamoxifen (in Canada) Novo-Tamoxifen (in Canada) PMS-Tamoxifen (in Canada) Tamofen (in Canada) Tamone (in Canada)	To treat breast cancer
Histamine H 2 Receptor Antagonists		Axid Mylanta AR Pepcid Tagamet Zantac	To treat duodenal ulcers, gastric ulcers, and conditions in which the stomach produces too much acid
Miscellaneous	Clofibrate	Abitrate Atromid-S Claripex (in Canada)	Used to lower cholesterol and triglyceride levels in the blood, control of seizures
	Primidone	Myidone Mysoline Apo-Primidone (in Canada) PMS Primidone (in Canada) Sertan (in Canada)	Anticonvulsant used to treat epilepsy and certain types of seizures

Resources

General Sexuality Resources

Many women have questions regarding the normality of their sexual thoughts, feelings, and behaviors. The resources listed in this section offer information about the range of women's sexual experiences. Many are based on large-scale surveys of women's (and sometimes men's) responses to interviews or questionnaires. The authors of these reports are experienced sex researchers or therapists. They offer their comments and insights in addition to statistics and information.

Ellison, Carol R. *Women's Sexualities: Generations of Women Share Intimate Secrets of Sexual Self-Acceptance.* Oakland, Calif.: New Harbinger Publications, 2000.
   Carol Ellison's book is based on a survey and interviews with 2,632 women between the ages of twenty and ninety! Dr. Ellison takes the approach that women of all ages can create their own erotic pleasure and sexual satisfaction. She offers some suggestions from her own clinical experience to help women do just that. The information in this book is highly relevant to women of all ages and is presented in a manner that stimulates insight and introspection into one's own sexual decisions and sexuality. It is a great companion book to *Reclaiming Your Sexual Self.*

Foley, Sallie, Sally A. Kope, and Dennis Sugrue. *Sex Matters for Women: A Complete Guide to Taking Care of Your Sexual Self.* New York: Guilford Press, 2002.
   This book was written by three experienced sex therapists and is based on their years of clinical experience. In it you will find a balanced discussion of the psychological and physical factors that contribute to women's sexual functioning, as well as advice on ways to make peace with your body, to create a better sexual relationship with your partner, and to overcome some common sexual difficulties. This book will be most relevant to you if your body image interferes with your sexual desire or if you or your partner has a sexual problem other than your low desire. There is an informative section in the book on male sexuality.

Michael, Robert T., John H. Gagnon, Edward O. Laumann, and Gina Kolata. *Sex in America: A Definitive Survey.* New York: Warner Books, 1995.
   If you have questions or concerns about what is normal, about how you compare with the general population, or about what other Americans are doing sexually, then

reading *Sex in America* will provide you with some answers. There are chapters on whom people partner with, how often they have sex, and what sexual activities they engage in, as well as chapters on trauma and sexually transmitted diseases. You will likely come away with the understanding that "normal" encompasses a wide range of sexual behaviors, but you may also get some information to challenge erroneous beliefs (yours and/or your partner's).

Books That Challenge the Status Quo on Female Sexuality

The history of medicine can be characterized by the study of men and the application of that study to women, whether appropriate or not. At last there are books that question the prevailing stereotypes and beliefs about women's sexuality. These thought-provoking books cannot fail to make you rethink some of your long-held notions of your own sexuality.

Angier, Natalie. *Woman: An Intimate Geography.* New York: Anchor Books, 1999.
This book confronts accepted stereotypes regarding women's anatomy and physiology and shows how cultural biases have influenced research and hence our understanding of what it is to be a woman. From the evolution of the clitoris to the story of the breast, from hormones to exercise to aggression—this wonderful book will make you examine your sexual and feminine self in a new way.

Kaschak, Ellyn, and Leonore Tiefer (eds.). *A New View of Women's Sexual Problems.* New York: Haworth Press, 2001.
This collection of essays by some of the leading feminist sex therapists and researchers disputes the medical model of female sexuality with its emphasis on proper genital functioning. *A New View* looks at a woman's sexual problems in the context of her life, her relationships, and the political and cultural climate in which she lives. This book will help women better understand the complexities behind their sexual complaints. With the current rush-to-market, magic-bullet medications for women's sexual disinterest, this book is essential reading. While some of the essays may be academic in tone, *A New View* is generally accessible to lay readers as well as professionals and students.

Orgasm for Women

One of the most frequent sexual complaints from women centers on the inability to achieve orgasm. Some women have difficulty experiencing orgasm regardless of whether they are by themselves or with a partner. Other women can have orgasms when they masturbate but are unable to climax when they are making love with their partner. The following books provide resources to help women understand and overcome orgasm problems.

Barbach, Lonnie. *For Yourself: The Fulfillment of Female Sexuality.* New York: Signet, 2000.

This book was originally published in 1976 and became a staple in the library of sex therapists. Dr. Barbach presents a series of exercises that are highly effective in helping most women achieve orgasm. This book is an excellent guide for women who have never or only rarely experienced orgasm. Its strength lies in the solo exercises, although there are some couples activities included as well.

Cattrall, Kim, and Mark Levinson. *Satisfaction: The Art of the Female Orgasm.* Boston: Warner Books, 2003.

This book was written for couples by a then husband-and-wife team. Kim Cattrall is an actress. Mark Levinson is a musician and music industry executive. While neither is a sex therapist, they bring their experiences as a sexually satisfied couple to the pages of this book. In easy-to-understand language and complete with diagrams, the authors outline simple techniques and sexual positions that will help promote sexual arousal and orgasm. As their own history attests, good sex alone does not make a good marriage, and there is little here that will address relationship or psychological issues. Nevertheless, this book is perhaps one of the most accessible guides to orgasm written for heterosexual partners.

Heiman, Julia R., and Joseph Lopiccolo. *Becoming Orgasmic: A Sexual and Personal Growth Program for Women,* New York: Fireside, 1992.

The title of this book is a bit of a misnomer. Although there is definitely help for women who want to experience orgasm, the book also discusses other sexual problems and touches on ways to enhance sexual pleasure. Written by two highly respected sex therapists and researchers, *Becoming Orgasmic* has information and advice for women of all ages.

Ladas, Alice K., Beverly Whipple, and John D. Perry. *The G Spot and Other Discoveries About Human Sexuality.* New York: Dell, 1983.

Don't let the date of this book fool you. It still has a lot of information that is very relevant for today. This groundbreaking book was the first to introduce the G-spot to female readers. It provides interesting background information about the rediscovery of this sensitive spot of female anatomy, but most important, this book gives women a greater understanding of orgasm and the variety of ways women experience it.

Winks, Cathy. *The Good Vibrations Guide: The G-Spot.* San Francisco: Down There Press, 1998.

This is an informative and readable book, which explains what the G-spot is and isn't. While presenting the anatomy and physiology, Cathy Winks also gives very practical advice on how to stimulate the G-spot to enhance sexual pleasure. The focus of this book is on discovering what turns you on and what doesn't. There is no performance demand here. While many women enjoy G-spot stimulation, many others don't, and there is no expectation that they should.

Sex Manuals

There are numerous sex manuals out there, and one can get truly overwhelmed by the vast selection. Sex is such a complex topic, and it is unlikely that one book will encompass it all. This is why it is best to refine your search, to look for books that address your particular concerns. Many sex books are written for people who want to spice up their sex lives. If you are looking for such books, the best idea is to read a few pages and see if you like the style and the information presented there. But if you have questions about basic techniques, or require accurate sexual information, you need to be choosier and pick books by professionals with some credentials or ones that are recommended by professionals.

Joannides, Paul. *Guide to Getting It On!* Waldport, Oregon: Goofy Foot Press, 2001.

This book is an informative, humorous, and straightforward sex guide. The author received input from a variety of people from all walks of life and has combined their anecdotes and quotes with explicit drawings and directions to provide everything from basic sex education (how to give a blow job) to sexual enhancement techniques (light bondage, fantasies, fetishes, sex toys). There is no better or no more comprehensive sex manual on the market today. A word of warning to those who cringe at sexually explicit and unscientific language: this book uses both.

Winks, Cathy, and Anne Semans. *The Good Vibrations Guide to Sex: The Most Complete Sex Manual Ever Written.* San Francisco: Cleis Press, 2002.

This is another very readable and informative sex guide that covers a wide range of topics. Quotations from real people and explicit line drawings give life to the sex information and advice contained within. There is a wealth of information about sex toys not available in other sex manuals.

Sexual Fantasy/Erotica

The ability to fantasize can be a powerful tool when you are attempting to reclaim your sexual desire. Many women feel guilty or ashamed of sexual fantasies and have had more practice repressing them rather than indulging in them. The books listed below are collections of erotica that may help you accept or expand your sexual imagination. If you don't currently fantasize but want to, these books can introduce you to the world of women's sexual fantasies and erotic writings. Women often find reading erotica more exciting than watching videos, and they may feel more comfortable buying a book and reading it than renting or buying an X-rated movie. Reading erotica can stimulate fantasy or help you to discover what turns you on (or off), and it can be a pleasure to experience alone or with your partner. These books are just suggestions. Please also look on the Web sites listed later in this section.

Barbach, Lonnie. *Pleasures: Women Write Erotica.* New York: Doubleday, 1984.

Bright, Susie (ed.). *Best American Erotica 2000.* New York: Touchstone Books, 2000.

Friday, Nancy. *My Secret Garden: Women's Sexual Fantasies.* New York: Pocket Books, 1974.

———. *Forbidden Flowers: More Women's Sexual Fantasies.* New York: Simon & Schuster, 1975.

Kudaka, Geraldine. *On a Bed of Rice: An Asian American Erotic Feast.* New York: Anchor, 1995.

Martin, Reginald (ed.). *Dark Eros: Black Erotic Writings.* New York: St. Martin's Press, 1997.

Queen, Carol, and Jack Davis (eds.). *Sex Spoken Here: Good Vibrations Erotic Reading Circle Selections.* San Francisco: Down There Press, 1998.

Sex and Motherhood

Raskin, Valerie. *Great Sex for Moms: Ten Steps to Nurturing Passion While Raising Kids.* New York: Fireside, 2002.

Dr. Raskin offers a "prescription" for staying passionate during parenthood that is divided into two phases: values and practical advice. The first part of the book examines the beliefs that women often hold as mothers and which interfere with their own pleasure (sexual and otherwise). The second part of the book contains some helpful advice on how to keep sex alive, but it is brief and of a general nature and is best read along with *Reclaiming Your Sexual Self* and *The Mother's Guide to Sex,* which is listed below.

Semans, Anne, and Cathy Winks. *The Mother's Guide to Sex.* New York: Three Rivers Press, 2001.

Semans and Winks take the reader on a journey from conception to parenting teenagers. *The Mother's Guide to Sex* affirms that sexuality is a part of our lives and our children's lives. It acknowledges the unique challenges posed by being both a mother and a sexual being and helps women navigate them more effectively. The pages of this book are filled with practical advice on how to have a pleasurable sex life despite having limited time, energy, privacy, and, often, resources.

Male Sexuality

It is always helpful to understand your male partner's sexuality and to confront some myths and misconceptions you may hold about his behavior. Reading books by men and about male sexuality can be extremely helpful and can also assist in opening the lines of communication between you and your partner. The recommended books in this section can be read by you or your partner, alone or together.

Milsten, Richard, and Julian Slowinski. *The Sexual Male: Problems and Solutions.* New York: W. W. Norton, 1999.

Written by a medical doctor and a psychologist who specialize in the treatment of sexual problems, this book looks at the array of sexual difficulties that can confront men at all stages of life. It may be of particular relevance if your partner is experiencing erection problems.

Zilbergeld, Bernie. *The New Male Sexuality: The Truth about Men, Sex, and Pleasure.* New York: Bantam Books, 1999.

This book examines the myths that many men hold about sex, performance, and women. It is easy to read, with many interesting and entertaining anecdotes. The book also provides very practical advice for dealing with some common sexual difficulties such as premature ejaculation and erection problems. The exercises can be done by your partner himself or with your help and cooperation.

Women's Health Issues

Reclaiming your sexual desire requires a healthy mind and body. The books in this section will provide you with information about how your body works, potential health problems, and the array of options you have to maintain your physical health. Any of the books in this section will provide you with additional information about many of the physical conditions that can affect your sexual desire.

Boston Women's Health Collective. *Our Bodies, Ourselves for the New Century: A Book by and for Women.* New York: Simon & Schuster, 1998.

Carlson, Karen J., Stephanie Eisenstat, and Terra Ziporyn. *The Harvard Guide to Women's Health.* Cambridge: Harvard University Press, 1996.

Siegal, Diana, and P. B. Doress. *New Ourselves, Growing Older.* New York: Simon & Schuster, 1996.

Northrup, Christiane. *Women's Bodies, Women's Wisdom.* New York: Bantam, 1998.

Menopause

Although there are many books on menopause available, this is the one book that I recommend you read. Dr. Northrup combines accurate medical information with a respect for the innate health and wisdom of women, to give us a new way of dealing with this change in our lives.

Northrup, Christiane. *The Wisdom of Menopause: Creating Physical and Emotional Health and Healing during the Change.* New York: Bantam Books, 2001.

This book covers a variety of topics that are important for women in midlife. These range from questions involving hormones, osteoporosis, cardiovascular disease, and breast cancer to information about sex, beauty, and vocational changes. Dr. Northrup helps women understand, respect, and deal with the changes their bodies are going through. Reading this book will help us find the balance between caring for ourselves and caring for others as we grow older. This balance is essential to maintaining sexual desire throughout life.

Exercise

Nelson, Miriam E. *Strong Women Stay Young*. New York: Bantam, 1998.

This positive and affirming book conveys the simple message that aging does not have to include physical weakness and deterioration. Dr. Nelson details an exercise program that every woman (no matter her age or physical condition) can follow. The exercises are well described and diagrammed. Dr. Nelson's own research shows that strength training (working out with weights) can turn back the clock and revitalize women physically and mentally. This is a wonderfully upbeat and inspiring book. If you have ever thought about starting an exercise program, or if you want to lose weight or have more energy, this is the book to read.

Sexual Abuse

Self-help books about abuse and trauma can provide much-needed validation for you as you heal. Reading about other women, their stories, and their recovery is tremendously empowering. The following books provide some help to bridge the transition to healthy sexuality once you have addressed the trauma in therapy.

Bass, Ellen, and Laura Davis. *The Courage to Heal*. New York: Perennial Press, 1994.

This groundbreaking book was the outgrowth of writing workshops for women, many of whom chose to write about their abuse. Much of the book is devoted to writing exercises designed to help women come to terms with the fact of their abuse. The book has been criticized on the grounds that it encourages women to believe they were abused even if they have no memory of abuse. It is not a good source for helping you resolve or understand feelings or symptoms you fear may spring from abuse you have no memory of. However, if you remember your abuse, this book can help you deal with the stigma and shame you may still carry with you. There is not a lot of help or information here on how to reclaim your sexuality; it is a resource best suited for women just beginning the healing process.

Haines, Staci. *The Survivor's Guide to Sex: How to Have an Empowered Sex Life After Child Sexual Abuse*. San Francisco: Cleis Press, 1999.

Maltz, Wendy. *The Sexual Healing Journey: A Guide for Survivors of Sexual Abuse*. New York: Harper Perennial, 1992.

——— and Beverly Holman. *Incest and Sexuality: A Guide to Understanding and Healing*. Lexington, Mass.: Lexington Books, 1987.

The four books listed above are excellent resources for women who have dealt with the trauma of sexual abuse (anxiety, flashbacks, depression) and are ready to address their sexuality. The books provide compassionate and sage advice for women beginning this sometimes difficult stage of the healing process.

Westerlund, Elaine. *Women's Sexuality After Childhood Incest*. New York: W. W. Norton, 1992.

This book provides a wealth of information regarding the effects of incest on adult sexuality in women. Based on the author's own research as well as on a review of other research in this area, it will help women to understand the various ways in which abuse can affect sexuality. There are two chapters devoted to treatment recommendations, which include a consideration of the impact of a woman's abuse on her partner. Despite the fact that this book is now somewhat dated, the information will still be relevant to many women.

Warshaw, Robin. *I Never Called It Rape: The Ms. Report on Recognizing, Fighting and Surviving Date and Acquaintance Rape.* New York: Harper Perennial, 1994.
This book presents statistics on the prevalence of date or acquaintance rape, which, though now ten years old, are still shocking. It will help women who experienced coercive sex to recognize the emotional impact that this experience has on them and their current partner.

For Partners of Abuse Survivors

It is very important that your partner understand and appreciate what you are going through as you heal from sexual abuse. It is also important that your partner be involved in the process, for his sake as well as yours. If you are involved in a relationship while you are dealing with the aftermath of sexual abuse, get one of the following books for you and your partner to read together. These books will help you maintain a positive connection with your partner while giving him some practical advice on how to both support you and deal with his own reactions.

Cameron, Grant. *What About Me? A Guide for Men Helping Female Partners Deal with Childhood Sexual Abuse.* Carp, Canada: Creative Bound, 1994.

Davis, Laura. *Allies in Healing: When the Person You Love Was Sexually Abused as a Child.* New York: Perennial Press, 1991.

Levine, Robert B. *When You Are the Partner of a Rape or Incest Survivor: A Workbook for You.* San Jose, Calif.: Resource Publications, 1996.

Alternative Therapies

Servan-Schreiber, David. *The Instinct to Heal: Curing Stress, Depression and Anxiety Without Drugs and Without Talk Therapy.* Emmaus, Penn.: Rodale, 2004.
Dr. Servan-Schreiber has written this informative book based on his experience as the co-founder of the University of Pittsburgh's Center for Complementary Medicine and his travels with the group Doctors Without Borders. Seven natural treatments for stress-related disorders are described as well as advice on how to integrate these therapies into your life. For anyone wanting to avoid medication for emotional disorders, this is a must-read book. Some of the therapies you can do on your own, others will require consulting a professional for help. There is a final section offering suggestions for improving communication in your personal relationships.

Communication

Gray, John. *Men Are from Mars, Women Are from Venus: A Practical Guide for Improving Communication and Getting What You Want in Your Relationships*. New York: HarperCollins, 1993.

While it contains some obvious oversimplifications and stereotyping, many men and women have found this book extraordinarily helpful in understanding and avoiding some common communication pitfalls. There is practical advice on how to more effectively convey your message to your partner. This book is written for both men and women.

Lerner, Harriet. *The Dance of Connection: How to Talk to Someone When You're Mad, Hurt, Scared, Frustrated, Insulted, Betrayed or Desperate*. New York: Quill, 2002.

The title of this book says it all. Dr. Lerner begins with helping us to understand that we learn how to communicate, which means that we can learn how to communicate differently and more effectively. She debunks many myths that are responsible for getting us stuck ("He has to apologize"; "I have to say what I feel") and offers us a new way of looking at relationships and new ways of communicating.

Tannen, Deborah. *You Just Don't Understand: Women and Men in Conversation*. New York: Ballantine, 1990.

Dr. Tannen is a professor of linguistics whose book highlights the complexities involved when men and women communicate. It will help you put your communication problems into a different perspective. While this is not a how-to book, it is unlikely that you will be able to talk to or listen to your partner in the same way again after reading it.

Relationships

Gottman, John, and Nan Silver. *The Seven Principles for Making Marriage Work*. New York: Three Rivers Press, 2000.

Based on Dr. Gottman's study of two thousand married couples, this book helps you evaluate the strengths and weaknesses of your marriage and gives you strategies and advice on how to improve it and strengthen its foundation. It's a very engaging book, with wonderful anecdotes and a series of self-tests that will get you thinking about your marriage in a constructive way.

Lerner, Harriet. *The Dance of Intimacy: A Woman's Guide to Courageous Acts of Change in Key Relationships*. New York: Perennial Press, 1997.

This book is a wonderful companion to *Reclaiming Your Sexual Self,* especially if your sexual desire problems reflect problems with intimacy. It acknowledges that becoming intimate is a process that defies simple techniques. Instead Dr. Lerner provides the reader with a foundation for thinking about and understanding intimacy that will help guide her as she engages with others. The importance of bringing a "self" to your relationships with others is clearly highlighted in this book.

Lerner, Harriet. *The Dance of Anger: A Woman's Guide to Changing the Patterns of Intimate Relationships.* New York: Quill, 2001.

In this book women are encouraged to listen to their anger and to use it constructively to build relationships. Another in the *Dance* series of books, this particular volume will be helpful to women whose low sexual desire is caused by unresolved anger. For women who are tired of the arguments about sex and are looking for a way to move beyond the fighting, this book will be invaluable.

McCann, Ellen. *The Two-Step: The Dance toward Intimacy.* New York: Grove Press, 1987.

A wonderful book that uses elegant drawings to illustrate the ways in which couples maintain distance in their relationships and the ways in which they can bridge the distance and achieve greater intimacy. It is a good book to share with your partner.

Domestic Violence

Jones, Ann, and Susan Schechter. *When Love Goes Wrong: What to Do When You Can't Do Anything Right.* New York: Harper Perennial, 1993.

Since all abuse is not physical, the first part of this book helps women determine if they are in an abusive relationship. For those who answer yes, the second part of the book is devoted to practical advice on how to safely get out of the relationship.

Infidelity

If you and your partner are interested in staying together in the aftermath of an affair, you will need some guidance. It is not enough simply to "put it behind you." Each of the following two books will help you understand the feelings of both partners and will walk you through the process of building trust again.

Brown, Emily M. *Affairs: A Guide to Working Through the Repercussions of Infidelity.* New York: Jossey-Bass, 1999.

Subotnik, Rona, and Gloria Harris. *Surviving Infidelity: Making Decisions, Recovering from the Pain.* Avon, Mass.: Adams, 1999.

Finding a Therapist

American Psychological Association
750 First Street N.E.
Washington, DC 20002-4242
Tel: (800) 374-2721/(202) 336-5500

Referral Information: (800) 964-2000
www.apa.org
The APA does not offer a referral service, but its Web site has links to state and provincial psychological associations that do. Try contacting your state or provincial association, or call (800) 964-2000 to locate the referral service in your area.

American Association for Marriage and Family Therapy
112 South Alfred Street
Alexandria, VA 22314-3061
Tel: (703) 838-9808
Fax: (703) 838-9805
www.aamft.org
The AAMFT does offer a referral service through its Web site. You may also contact its main office.

American Association of Sex Educators, Counselors and Therapists (AASECT)
See listing below.

Organizations and Web Sites— Sexual Information

American Association of Sex Educators, Counselors and Therapists (AASECT)
P.O. Box 5488
Richmond, VA 23220-0488
Tel: (804) 644-3288
www.aasect.org
This organization provides a certification for sex therapists. In addition to helping you locate a therapist among one of its certified members, AASECT provides a list of books and articles by members and links to other sexuality Web sites.

The Kinsey Institute for Research in Sex, Gender and Reproduction
313 Morrison Hall
Indiana University
Bloomington, IN 47405
Tel: (812) 855-7686
www.kinseyinstitute.org
The Web site provides sexuality information links. The Kinsey Institute also operates a clinic for the treatment of sexual problems.

The New View Campaign
163 Third Avenue
PMB#183
New York, NY 10003
Tel: (212) 533-2774
Fax: (212) 254-5922
www.fsd-alert.org

New View is an educational campaign to challenge the myths promoted by the pharmaceutical industry. The Web site provides information and resources regarding relevant issues.

Planned Parenthood
Tel: (800) 230-7526
www.plannedparenthood.org
The Web site will help you locate a Planned Parenthood office near you. The site also offers health information related to contraception and sexuality.

Sexuality Information and Education Council of the United States (SIECUS)
130 West 42nd Street, Suite 350
New York, NY 10036
Tel: (212) 819-9770
www.siecus.org
SIECUS develops, collects, and disseminates sexuality information and promotes sex education. Information and resources are available for adults, teens, schools, and organizations.

Society for Sexuality
www.sexuality.org
A sex education Web circle comprised of select Web sites, each of which offers a unique and free contribution to Internet sex education.

Organizations and Web Sites—Menopause

American Menopause Foundation
350 Fifth Avenue, Suite 2822
New York, NY 10118
Tel: (212) 714-2398
www.americanmenopause.org
The AMF provides information and resources for women regarding menopause.

North American Menopause Society
P.O. Box 94527
Cleveland, OH 44101
Tel: (440) 442-7550
Fax: (440) 442-2660
Automated consumer request line: (800) 774-5342
E-mail: info@menopause.org
www.menopause.org
The NAMS provides information on menopause to health care providers and the public.

Organizations and Web Sites—STDs

American Social Health Association—Herpes/HIV ResourceCenter
P.O. Box 13827
Research Triangle Park, NC 27709
Tel: (800) 230-6039
National Herpes Hotline: (919) 361-8488
www.ashastd.org

Centers for Disease Control and Prevention
National STD Hotline: (800) 227-8922
www.CDC.gov

Hepatitis Information Network (Hepnet)
Tel: (800) 223-0179
www.hepnet.com

National HIV/AIDS Hotline
Tel: (800) 342-AIDS (in English); (800) 344-7432 (in Spanish)

Organizations and Web Sites—Sexual Pain

International Pelvic Pain Association
Tel: (205) 877-2950 or (800) 624-9676
www.pelvicpain.org

National Vulvodynia Association
P.O. Box 4491
Silver Spring, MD 20914-4491
Tel: (301) 299-0775
Fax: (301) 299-3999
www.nva.org

University of Michigan Center for Vulvar Disease
University of Michigan Health System
1500 E. Medical Center Drive
Ann Arbor, MI 48109
Tel: (734) 763-6295
www.med.umich.edu/obgyn/vulva

Vulvar Pain Foundation
P.O. Drawer 177
Graham, NC 27253

Tel: (336) 226-0704
Fax: (336) 226-8518
www.vulvarpainfoundation.org

Organizations and Web Sites—Domestic Violence and Sexual Abuse

National Domestic Violence Hotline
Tel: (800)799-SAFE or 1-800-787-3224 (TTY)
    Provides information and referrals across the United States.
    www.ndvh.org

VOICES in Action, Inc.
8041 Hosbrook, Suite 236
Cincinnati, OH 45236
Tel: (800) 7-VOICE8
www.voices-action.org
    VOICES promotes education and awareness regarding the impact and prevalence of child sexual abuse. This organization provides support to adult victims and organizes yearly conferences for its members.

Erotica and Sex Toys

The stores and Web sites listed here are run by women. They are tastefully presented and, while sexually explicit, are not pornographic. Visiting these sites will not result in a deluge of pornographic spam, which often happens with other online sex shops.

Good Vibrations
938 Howard Street, Suite 101
San Francisco, CA 94103
Tel: (415) 974-8990/(800) 289-8423
www.goodvibes.com

Toys in Babeland (TIB)
www.babeland.com
    Toys in Babeland also has workshops on various sex-related topics in their stores. Some recent workshops have dealt with sex toys, the G spot, and an introduction to S&M.

TIB Lower East Side
94 Rivington Street

New York, NY 10002
Tel: (212) 375-1701

TIB Soho
43 Mercer Street
New York, NY 10013
Tel: (212) 966-2120

TIB Seattle
707 E. Pike Street
Seattle, WA 98122
Tel: (206) 328-2914

Index

"This interesting and eminently readable book comes at a critical time for women pressured to seek chemical solutions to low sexual desire. Dr. Hall helps women to understand what causes and maintains low desire and suggests various solutions through a series of practical exercises. The book contains a wealth of information that will empower women to "reclaim" and not "blame" themselves."

—Lana Stermac, Ph.D., Professor, Counseling Psychology Program, Ontario Institute for Studies in Education, University of Toronto

"Highly, highly, highly recommended for everyone, not just women with wow desire. Kathryn Hall is an excellent sex therapist and she treats low desire as a messenger rather than as a disease. Men and women both will be able to find approaches in her book that can help them better understand and give meaning to lost desire. She believes that low desire means different things to different people, and she presents a number of ways of approaching it. Fortunately, she is not beholden to the drug companies and realizes the short-sightedness of automatically throwing pills or patches at whatever ails you."

—Paul Joannides, author of *Guide To Getting It On,* 4th Edition

"Dr. Hall begins with the fundamental premise that our sexual self is much more than the sum of our biological parts. Not surprisingly, then, her book is an intelligent and frank presentation of the personal and interpersonal forces that shape our sexual interest and desire and the effective strategies for their control. A must read for every woman who wishes to understand better this important aspect of her identity. Indeed, the many who are searching for sexual desire in an easy-to-swallow pill form may be pleasantly surprised to find it in this easy-to-read book form."

—Gerianne M. Alexander, Ph.D., Assistant Professor of Psychology, Texas A&M University

"Everyone needs to be informed about sexuality. A wonderful sex life comes no more automatically than a wonderful trip to Paris. Preparation can help people find the good parts and deal with problems. Dr. Hall's book is addressed to women who feel they have problems with sexual desire and it includes many vignettes, suggestions, exercises for reflection, further references, and excellent insights based on her experience as a sex therapist. I will recommend this book to my patients.

—Leonore Tiefer, Ph.D., Clinical Associate Professor of Psychiatry, New York University School of Medicine

Printed in the USA
CPSIA information can be obtained
at www.ICGtesting.com
JSHW022324140824
68134JS00019B/1281